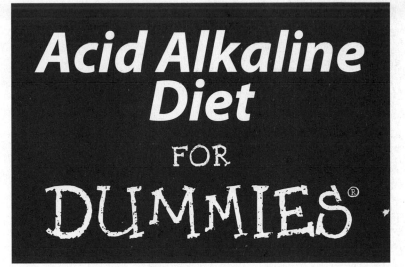

Acid Alkaline Diet FOR DUMMIES®

by Julie Wilkinson, RN, BSN

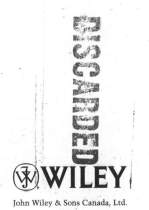

WILEY

John Wiley & Sons Canada, Ltd.

Acid Alkaline Diet For Dummies®

Published by
John Wiley & Sons Canada, Ltd.
6045 Freemont Blvd.
Mississauga, ON L5R 4J3

www.wiley.com

For general information on John Wiley & Sons Canada, Ltd., including all books published by Wiley Publishing, Inc., please call our warehouse, Tel 1-800-567-4797. For reseller information, including discounts and premium sales, please call our sales department, Tel 416-646-7992. For press review copies, author interviews, or other publicity information, please contact our marketing department, Tel 416-646-4584, Fax 416-236-4448.

For technical support, please visit www.wiley.com/techsupport.

Wiley publishes in a variety of print and electronic formats and by print-on-demand. Some material included with standard print versions of this book may not be included in e-books or in print-on-demand. If this book refers to media such as a CD or DVD that is not included in the version you purchased, you may download this material at http://booksupport.wiley.com. For more information about Wiley products, visit www.wiley.com.

Library and Archives Canada Cataloguing in Publication Data

Wilkinson, Julie

    Acid alkaline diet for dummies / Julie Wilkinson.

Includes index.

ISBN 978-1-118-41418-7 (pbk); ISBN 978-1-118-41419-4 (e-PDF); ISBN 978-1-118-41420-0 (e-Mobi); ISBN 978-1-118-41421-7 (e-Pub)

    1. Acid-base imbalances–Diet therapy. 2. Acid-base

imbalances–Nutritional aspects. 3. Diet therapy. I. Title.

RM216.W54 2012   615.8'54   C2012-906676-1

Printed in the United States

1 2 3 4 5 RRD 16 15 14 13 12

About the Author

Julie Wilkinson (RN, BSN) is a patient advocate and active Registered Nurse who has achieved multiple commendations throughout her career, including a Meritorious Achievement Medal for Civilian Service and Civilian Nurse of the Year from the Department of Defense. When she is not providing bedside patient care and education, she is the Guide to Colon Cancer on About.com and writes for a number of health and well-being publications as a freelancer, including LiveSTRONG.com.

Dedication

This book is dedicated to my two beautiful sons, James and Jack, who are truly a blessing. You are the best children a mother could ever hope for — thank you so much for being such good boys. I owe my strong foundation and wordsmith capabilities to my late parents, who I know would be ecstatic to see this book in print. I'd also like to dedicate it to my husband and my entire family for their support and inexhaustible encouragement.

Author's Acknowledgments

I'd like to start with Kathleen Dobie, my project editor. Thank you so much for walking me through this process. Your emails, support, and attitude made collaboration very enjoyable. A big thank you for taking my thoughts and ideas and helping me turn them into a presentable, readable text.

Thank you Anam Ahmed, my project manager, for presenting me with this opportunity and entrusting me to write your vision. The enthusiasm you've shown for this book was contagious.

Thank you Allison Tannis, the technical reviewer of this book, as well as the recipe tester, Emily Nolan, and nutritional analyst, Patty Santelli, who had their hands full with my culinary visions.

Finally, I want to include everyone at John Wiley & Sons who was involved with this project. The editors, production staff, artists — I may not know each of you by name, but your hard work is what takes a bunch of words and turns them into an engaging, finished product.

Publisher's Acknowledgments

We're proud of this book; please send us your comments at http://dummies.custhelp.com. For other comments, please contact our Customer Care Department within the U.S. at 877-762-2974, outside the U.S. at 317-572-3993, or fax 317-572-4002.

Some of the people who helped bring this book to market include the following:

Acquisitions and Editorial

Project and Copy Editor: Kathleen Dobie

Acquisitions Editor: Anam Ahmed

Technical Editor: Allison Tannis

Recipe Tester: Emily Nolan

Nutritional Analyst: Patty Santelli

Production Editor: Lindsay Humphreys

Editorial Assistant: Kathy Deady

Cover Photo: © River Albu / iStock

Back Cover Photos: © Zlatko Kostic / iStock
© Elena Elisseeva / iStock

Cartoons: Rich Tennant (www.the5thwave.com)

Composition Services

Project Coordinator: Kristie Rees

Layout and Graphics: Jennifer Creasey, Christin Swinford

Proofreaders: John Greenough, Wordsmith Editorial

Indexer: Estalita Slivoskey

John Wiley & Sons Canada, Ltd.

Deborah Barton, Vice President and Director of Operations

Jennifer Smith, Vice President and Publisher, Professional Development

Alison Maclean, Managing Editor, Professional Development

Publishing for Consumer Dummies

Kathleen Nebenhaus, Vice President and Executive Publisher

Composition Services

Debbie Stailey, Director of Composition Services

Contents at a Glance

Recipes at a Glance

Table of Contents

Introduction

*E*very living creature has a *pH balance,* which is a delicate balance of acid and alkaline chemicals. The human body is designed to be slightly *alkaline* — to have a pH slightly higher than 7. If you eat foods that drop your pH, or makes it acidic, your body goes into DEFCON 4 to bring it back to its normal, alkaline state.

Everything you do affects your pH. The good news? You can help your body control your pH through diet, which sets the stage for health and longevity. By eating a balanced acid alkaline diet, you take the extra work from your body so it can get back to its primary purpose — keeping you alive and well.

Although it's not a common household term, the acid alkaline diet has been around for a long time. To some people, eating a pH balanced diet to improve wellness is synonymous with chin piercing and poodles wearing velour jumpsuits. In a word, they think it's weird. However, they're probably already eating a similar diet and calling it by its more common name, which is simply *eating healthy*.

Unless you leave your pH urine test strips on the counter, there's nothing weird or alternative about this diet. Despite all the gimmicks surrounding pH dieting, the central concept is pretty straightforward — you eat foods that naturally help your body function at its best.

About This Book

Whether you're reading this book because you already have an illness or you're reading it because you want to stay healthy, you're holding 24 chapters packed with everything you need to get started on a pH balanced diet and lifestyle.

Carnivore, omnivore, herbivore, vegetarian — it doesn't really matter what you were before you picked up *Acid Alkaline Diet For Dummies*. You — and everyone you know — can fit this diet into your life and improve your potential for health without counting every calorie and spending hundreds of dollars on specialty foods.

I don't throw lists at you and tell you what you can and cannot eat. I show you why your body needs a specific blend of both acid- and alkaline-forming foods. You also see why certain foods and beverages are better for you and how to incorporate them into your diet — anytime and anyplace.

Conventions Used in This Book

Depending on where you jump in, you may notice that I use the words *acid, acidifying,* and *acid-forming* interchangeably. They mean the same thing and describe a substance that makes your pH *more acidic.*

Likewise, I also refer to any substances that turn the body more alkaline as *alkaline-forming, alkalinizing,* and *base* substances.

The following are some additional conventions to make your reading more pleasurable:

✔ This book contains some words that may be unfamiliar. I've placed these words in *italics* and they're followed with a definition.

✔ Keywords or things that I think are vital to understanding the diet are in **boldface**.

✔ Web sites are typed exactly as I found them in monofont. If a Web address needed to break across two lines of text during the printing process, rest assured that there are no any extra characters (such as hyphens) to indicate the break. So, when using one of these Web addresses, just type in exactly what you see in this book, pretending the line break doesn't exist.

Foolish Assumptions

I'm guessing you sought out this book because you want to start eating a healthy pH balanced diet. That was my main assumption while I wrote it. I worked to impart the acid alkaline know-how without providing a full-on biochemistry lesson about pH and the body. I'm not a doctor or nutritionist, and I don't play one on TV. I'm a registered nurse who has helped hundreds of people learn how to balance nutrition and lifestyle to promote health.

Another safe assumption: It's a food book, so it has recipes. I provide four full chapters of acid-alkaline-balanced recipes that have been taste-tested on real people (other than my family).

Last assumption. I don't have a big white hat and bachelor's degree in culinary arts, and chances are, you don't either. Perfect! The balanced recipes I provide may not end up in a five-star restaurant, but they are delicious and simple.

What You're Not to Read

One of the best things about the *For Dummies* books is their proclivity for extraneous information. I put this information in something called *sidebars,* which are the grayed-out boxes of text. You don't have to read them if you don't want to, and they won't impact your diet success. Other scientific tidbits are marked with a Technical Stuff icon. Again, skip 'em if you're in a rush to get pH balanced.

How This Book is Organized

Acid Alkaline Diet For Dummies is organized into seven different parts ranging from practical to yummy to scientific. Feel free to skip around if that's how you process information! In the meantime, following is a summary of what you can find in each part.

Part 1: Acid Alkaline Basics

If you've already started researching the diet, then you've probably come across conflicting (and frustrating!) information on the web. pH diets are largely misunderstood, with new web pages sprouting up daily to sell alkaline products. Unlike those web pages, this part introduces the concept of acid alkaline dieting without any pop-ups or ads.

I explain how to identify acid-forming versus alkaline-forming foods, allowing you to be self-sufficient in the grocery store and in restaurants. After all, who wants a list of foods to eat and not to eat stapled to their forehead? (If you do, there may be a *Piercing Addictions For Dummies* book available.)

Part I also includes pH testing methods and instruction for the scientific-minded folk. It's a fun and inexpensive way to track your pH, but not completely essential.

Part II: Homeostasis: Keeping Your Body Happy

Okay, so what the heck is homeostasis and who cares? Homeostasis is a fancy word that describes the way your body keeps itself balanced and alive. This part includes the background on how the acid alkaline diet works. When you understand that everything you do — and don't do — impacts your pH, you're better prepared to manage it.

The chapters in this part illustrate all of the things that impact your pH. I wish I could say that diet alone can keep your body alkaline, but it's just not true. Exercise, alcohol, and even your mood have the potential to make your body acidic, which sets the stage for disease.

Part III: Making the Switch: Starting Your Diet

Ready, set, get cooking! Even if you've never picked up a spatula, Part III is designed to help you prepare, shop, and stock up for success on the acid alkaline diet. It also covers why all those convenience-type meals are saturated in acid-forming ingredients and need to go bye-bye.

I realize that some of you may have an illness — hence the desire to want to eat healthier foods and help your body heal. This part contains valuable information about addressing your doctor and other health professionals as well as how some pills and supplements can adversely impact your pH.

Part IV: Let's Eat!

Eyes of newt and wings of bat . . . okay, okay, I promise there's nothing scary in Part IV. I know it's extremely off putting to pick up a healthy cookbook and find nothing you recognize on the ingredients list. With a few tiny exceptions, you should recognize (and be able to pronounce) all of the ingredients in the recipes in this part.

Whether it's breakfast or a midnight snack, Part IV contains dozens of recipes that are tasty and good for your pH. You won't have a hard time following my instructions, even if you hate to cook.

Part V: Overcoming Obstacles to Your pH Goals

We all get stuck in a rut from time to time — it's human nature! Part V gives you the tools to dig yourself out, no matter what your excuse may be. Business lunch meeting? Got it covered in Chapter 18. Upcoming big food holiday? Coping strategies are laid out in Chapter 19. Spouse unwilling to embrace the diet? Chapter 21 offers encouragement and suggestions. Find helpful tips for keeping your body balanced in any situation, including a whole chapter on weight loss challenges — that's Chapter 20, in this part.

Part VI: The Part of Tens

I can't take credit for this one. Part VI is a traditional *For Dummies* must-read (and is probably the most dog-eared portion of the book). I think of it as the most helpful part of the book, where you can find the bottom line on the best and the worst things you can do for your pH balance in three succinct chapters.

Part VII: Appendixes

If the book's a cake, this part would be the frosting. You don't have to read them, but both appendixes provide useful information that can help you along your journey to a balanced pH. The first appendix is a reference tool, providing pages of substitutes to help you exchange acid-forming foods and ingredients for more alkaline-friendly choices. The second appendix includes a metric conversion chart, which helps everyone speak the same language in the kitchen.

Icons Used in This Book

You may want to take a look at the icons listed here. These neat little pictures are sprinkled throughout the book to draw attention to the text they're next to. What they draw attention to and how important that info is to you, I'll leave for you to decide.

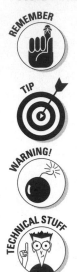

Watch out for these. I use them to mark information that bears repeating.

This icon points to handy information that can help you balance your pH without enduring common pitfalls.

Pay close attention to text marked with this icon. It highlights potentially dangerous mistakes on the diet.

This icon represents scientific info or a fun fact. The info next to this icon isn't strictly necessary for understanding the topic at hand.

Where to Go from Here

What do you want to know about? If you're just dying to take a peek at the recipes, head to Part IV. Do you want to start testing your pH? Chapter 4 explains how to do that. Wherever you want to go is fine with me! Just flip to the section that calls to you and start reading. This book is meant to help you find out about the acid alkaline diet, not force you to read through from page one to the end. (I don't teach 6th grade chemistry and I'm not going to quiz you!)

I do have one teeny piece of advice. If you know nothing of pH or how your body works, it may help to start with Chapter 5. It provides the basics of pH and a very light-hearted overview of how your body works to maintain it.

Part I
Getting to Know the Basics

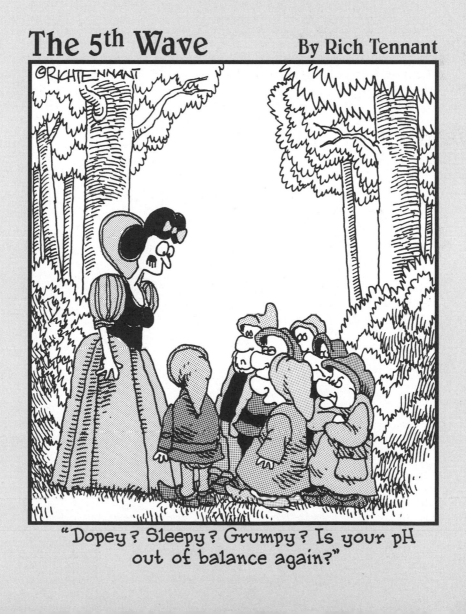

The 5th Wave   By Rich Tennant

"Dopey? Sleepy? Grumpy? Is your pH
out of balance again?"

In this part...

The acid alkaline diet is quite often misunderstood. Foods are not acidifying or alkalinizing based on their inherent pH — that's where the majority of people get it wrong. Foods are acid *forming* or alkaline *forming* dependant on their mineral content during digestion.

This part provides an introduction to those foods and shows how they can adversely affect every system in your body. An acid build-up is no more than a stockpile of waste. Left unchecked, this waste can lead to disease and destruction. If the proof truly is in the pudding, you'll see this for yourself after I show you how to test your body's pH at the end of this part. It's a fairly inexpensive way to show that you really are what you eat.

Chapter 1

Rebooting Your Body

In This Chapter

▶ Discovering how a pH balanced diet works

▶ Uncovering the mysteries shrouding acid alkaline diets

▶ Realizing simple changes make a big difference

▶ Reviewing the benefits of diet and lifestyle changes

*E*ver wish you could start all over again (skipping puberty, of course)? To be in a state of perfect wellness, unpolluted by years of fast food, preservatives, and other chemicals? Whether your arteries are clogged or your gallbladder went on strike years ago, it's not too late to make a change and grab your health by the horns.

What do you do when technology acts up? Most of us hit the power switch and reboot the device (while cursing it). When you flick it back on, 99.9 percent of the time, the problem's fixed.

Wouldn't it be amazing if you had a reboot button? Imagine what that would be like . . . Oops, ate too many saturated fats this week . . . hit reboot on the cardiovascular system. Celebrated a winning softball game with five slices of meat-lovers pizza. No problem, just reboot the gastrointestinal tract. Fact is, there's a way to reboot your body. You can start right now. Today. This instant. Put down that soda and keep reading. You are not enslaved to your past. Start making better choices today to impact your health tomorrow.

Revealing the Acid Alkaline Diet

The acid alkaline diet has a number of nicknames including the "*Miracle Diet*," "*pH Diet*," and simply the "*Alkaline Diet*," but they all refer to the same nutritional technique: balancing acid and alkaline foods for health.

Following a pH-balancing, acid alkaline diet is one of the best things you can do for your health. Don't take my word for it, look at the stacks of scientific evidence. The results of many peer-reviewed studies, including one published in 2007 by the Human Nutrition Research Center, prove that diets rich in alkaline-forming foods provide myriad health benefits. Focusing on elderly diets, the same study found that alkaline foods, including fresh vegetables, helped the elderly combat acids in dietary proteins and improve their ability to retain healthy muscle mass. Mom knew what she was talking about when she told you to eat your veggies!

Acid-forming foods are bad for you. But you may not realize the danger , because the damage starts inside, where you can't see it. Out of sight, out of mind — sadly, that's how many view their diet-health connection. They can't see the damage acid-forming foods are causing, so they don't do anything to change it.

On an acid alkaline diet you see the results of the foods you eat when you measure your pH. These measurements reflect the acid-alkaline balance in your body.

Okay, what are acids and alkalines?

Everything in the universe has an opposing force — night and day, yin and yang, and, of course, acid and alkaline. On a linear 0 to 14 pH scale, acidic substances (think stomach acid) range from the lowest pH of 0 to 7. Vinegar, for instance, has a pH reading of about 2.0 (acidic). Conversely, alkaline substances (think minerals) fall between 7 and 14 on the scale. Calcium, which is highly alkaline, has a pH around 10.

Every food (and drink) you ingest has the potential to form acid or alkaline *ash* during digestion. This leftover slush of chemicals has the potential to alter your body's pH environment, which is how foods are categorized as "acid forming" or "alkaline forming." I talk more about that in Chapters 2 and 5. For now, the takeaway is that pretty much everything you eat and drink impacts your pH balance, which impacts your health.

Balancing your pH

An acid alkaline diet doesn't require fancy supplements or prepackaged meals. The whole point is to help your body balance its *pH*, which is the overall measurement of acids and bases (also called alkalines) throughout your body. Your body is naturally alkaline (pH greater than 7.0) and functions at its best when it's more alkaline. However, chronically eating acid-forming foods (think red meat) tips your pH balance out of whack and sets the stage for illness.

We should know better by now

In the American northeast, nestled in the woods of Beltsville, Maryland, lies the Beltsville Human Nutrition Research Center. Their claim to fame is that they were the first facility to compile a research study detailing the effects of diet and nutrition in humans. According to their website, this occurred around the 1890s.

By the 20th century, even Samuel Clemens, more widely known as Mark Twain (1835-1910), knew about diet and health publications as evidenced by his famous quote, "Be careful about reading health books. You may die of a misprint."

Now, in the 21st century, we have almost too much information at our fingertips, yet we continue to pollute our systems with unpronounceable chemicals, fatty foods, and acids. I don't know about you, but I intend to pay attention to three centuries of research.

Today, everyone knows that dietary choices impact the human body in myriad ways and that poor food choices lead to disease. Now is the time to start doing something about it. Check out Chapter 3 for more information on the impacts of diet on health.

Your pH balance influences every single function in your body, from breathing to digestion. You have the ability to influence your pH through diet and lifestyle by making more alkaline choices.

Ignoring the unenlightened

During your journey to pH balance, you may come across people — colleagues, friends, even family members — who either don't understand the acid alkaline diet or openly preach that it's a fraudulent fad. I implore you to keep this thought in the back of your mind at all times:

How can eating a diet composed largely of natural vegetables, fruits, and lean proteins not have excellent outcomes? Day-glow orange socks and jelly bracelets are fads; eating for your health is not.

If I told you to cut out an entire food group, don a purple tutu, or severely restrict your daily calories — now that's weird. There's nothing weird or alternative about eating to influence your health. It's scientific fact that acidic foods leach minerals from your body and can negatively impact your state of wellness. I'm going to show you how to drop some of those acids (the purple tutu's optional).

Taking Charge of Your pH

Yes, you can control your pH balance, as well as how hard your body has to work to keep it in check. If you're constantly putting acids in your body, it's constantly working to remove said acids and doesn't have time for much else.

Acids in your body are like a poorly behaved five year old in the grocery store. He's running down the aisles tipping soda bottles over and dumping displays of food. Your body, (the store clerk) is constantly pulling a "clean up on Aisle 7" routine. With all that extra work, the clerk doesn't have time to restock shelves, place orders, or care for the general upkeep of the store. It's time to take charge of your pH and stop letting the five year old run amuck.

Making better choices

Sounds simple, right? It is. Working toward a healthy, balanced pH is as straightforward as choosing a carrot over a puffed orange crunchie. Although I demonstrate how to check urine pH measurements, keep logs, and even make shopping lists, you don't have to do any of that to enjoy the benefits of being more alkaline today than you were yesterday.

Your success on the acid alkaline diet boils down to choice — you can fill three-quarters of your plate with fresh vegetables or with processed foods. The vegetables contain vitamins, fiber, and alkalinizing minerals, whereas the processed food contains acidifying chemicals, fatty acids, cholesterol, and probably excessive calories and sodium. Your choice.

Altering your diet

You will have to alter what you eat on the acid alkaline diet, but you won't have to go crazy and donate half the food in your fridge to local shelters. I don't want you to pretend you can permanently abstain from your comfort foods — that almost always leads to giving up on a diet.

Instead, there are ways to minimize these comfort foods — while still enjoying them — and make alkaline-forming foods the star on your plate. I explain the basics of what you can eat plenty of and which foods to restrict or eliminate in Chapter 11.

Some diets are so restrictive you're scared to even go to a restaurant. Never fear, your pH guru's here. Chapters 18 and 19 cover dining out, holidays, and even enjoying special occasions while still adhering to an alkaline lifestyle.

Making Healthy Food Choices

Soon you'll understand how to differentiate when it's safe to tell your inner five year old "no" and when you can say "yes." He's going to sit on your shoulder and beg for a grilled cheese, a cold glass of milk, and a helping of French fries. You don't have to quit eating everything you enjoy, you just need to discover how to select more alkaline-forming foods and fill your plate with them.

What I'm encouraging you to eat

The purpose of eating more alkaline-forming foods is twofold:

- ✔ You decrease the amount of acid-forming foods you munch on, which allows your body to take a break from correcting your pH and focus on general housekeeping — boosting your immune system, recovering from disease or illness, and so on.

- ✔ A consistently alkaline pH allows your body to start fixing acid build-up and all of the health problems associated with it, such as digestive disorders or skin problems. Now that you're no longer bombarding your body with acids, it can focus on healing itself and repairing damage.

Alkaline-forming foods are synonymous with healthy foods and include:

- ✔ Vegetables
- ✔ Fruits (natural, not sweetened or dried)
- ✔ Sprouted grains
- ✔ Almonds and lentils
- ✔ Tofu and soy products

If you're hankering to see a list of what you should and shouldn't eat (although I don't recommend such a restrictive mindset), you'll find one in Chapter 11.

What I'm discouraging you from eating

You should limit the acid-forming foods to encompass between 20 and 40 percent of your plate, tops. Acid-forming foods come in shades of gray — you have a choice of lean animal proteins (poultry), that are the least acid-forming, and you have the atomic bomb of acid proteins, which are your fatty red meats and wild game. Some examples of the acid-forming foods include:

> ✔ Red and processed meats
>
> ✔ Fried and fatty foods
>
> ✔ Whole dairy products
>
> ✔ Yeasty breads and wheat products
>
> ✔ Sugar-laden snacks and beverages

Although these foods should be limited, you can enjoy the occasional sweet treat or fatty morsel. I show you how to balance them with a healthy diet in Chapter 2.

Finding hidden acids

Take a walk to your pantry. Do you see ketchup, mayonnaise, salad dressings, croutons, and coffee? They're what I like to call the *hidden acids,* and each of them impacts your pH in a bad way. I could proclaim myself a health freak because I had a piece of toast for breakfast, salad for lunch, and chicken breast for dinner. What I forgot to mention was the fact that my toast was smothered in jelly, my salad was awash in ranch-style dressing, and my chicken breast was fried — all of a sudden it's not so healthy when you take off the rose-colored glasses.

These tiny, seemingly inconsequential hidden acids add up! Acid-forming foods are acid-forming foods — no matter the size. Take a piece of broccoli and drench it in cheese sauce. You just nixed the alkaline-forming potential of that amazing vegetable. Don't render your alkaline-forming foods null and void; embrace their natural flavors, and leave the sauces, gravies, and condiments to someone else.

How Food and Life Impact pH

Your health is a long-term investment. I know it sounds really easy for me to sit here saying, "quit doing (insert bad habit here)." I realize that habits, such as tobacco use, poor dietary choices, or even a sedentary lifestyle, are very hard to break. But I didn't say impossible, did I? Chapter 6 explains how you can start improving your pH lifestyle one habit at a time.

The human body maintains a slightly alkaline pH, sometimes to your detriment. If acids are running amuck in your system, your body leeches calcium and other minerals from your bones to neutralize them. Rather than letting your acidic pH balance treat your bones like an ATM for calcium, it's better to cut out some of the acid-forming substances in your life.

I realize this is a diet book, but any well-rounded diet worth its salt should also address your behavior outside of food choices. Picking and eating the right foods won't get you all the way to the finish line. You have to alter some behaviors as well.

Some lifestyle-acquired acids that can ruin your pH include:

- ✔ Smoking and tobacco use
- ✔ Drinking alcohol
- ✔ Leading a sedentary life
- ✔ Overdoing the workouts
- ✔ Ingesting coffee, soda, and other stimulants
- ✔ Using recreational drugs
- ✔ Being consistently dehydrated (not drinking enough water)

Reversing the Damage

The human body has an almost miraculous ability to heal, but only if you give it the right tools. Instead of rationalizing poor choices by saying the damage's already done, you can use that energy to power a lifestyle and dietary change aimed toward wellness.

For every ten men or women diagnosed with a dietary-impacted illness (diabetes, high blood pressure, and anemia, for example), I'd bet over half of them didn't change their lifestyle or diet after diagnosis. Many illnesses can be halted, if not reversed, through diet alone.

Taking baby steps

Change one thing in favor of your pH balance, or change absolutely everything — it's up to you. But experts agree that taking small steps toward a goal is the best way to reach it.

Years ago I tried a diet where I basically had to ditch all my favorite comfort foods. Tracking calories, ounces, and macronutrients was required at every meal and snack. I had lists of "good" foods and "bad" ones. I can't tell you whether the diet was beneficial or not because it lasted all of two weeks.

I don't encourage you to come that far out of your comfort zone. If the recipes with tofu freak you out, avoid them. If you faint at the site of vegetables, start by cutting some acid-forming foods out of your diet (red meats, sodas). Then, you can build on that small but sturdy foundation one step at a time.

Tracking changes

Tracking your pH measurements may help illustrate your results. I can't predict when you'll start seeing results from a balanced pH diet, nor could anyone. But if you put pen to paper and start tracking those daily morning pH results (as well as how you feel), you can see the changes for yourself. It's a relatively cheap process, and I tell you how to test in Chapter 4.

Embracing Health

Sometimes you simply make bad dietary choices — on purpose. You know you should've avoided that jelly-filled donut, but you wanted it. Embracing health can be as easy as understanding that for every dietary choice you make, there's a reaction in your body — good or bad. It's a little more complicated than eat grilled pickles and get diarrhea, but the concept's similar.

Some of the ways an acid alkaline balanced diet can help you improve your health include:

✔ Increased fiber in your diet leads to a healthier colon, decreased cholesterol, increased weight control, and manageable blood sugars.

✔ Decreased saturated fats promotes a healthier cardiovascular system (heart, arteries), easier weight control, and a decreased risk of stroke.

✔ Increased nutrients gives your body the right tools — vitamins, minerals, and phytochemicals — to function as it was meant to.

So there's no potion, pill, or device you need to enjoy an acid alkaline diet — just healthy foods!

It's absolutely heartbreaking when it does occur, but, fortunately chronic diseases are not as common in children as they are in their adult counterparts. This is because they've not polluted their little bodies yet — they're still functioning on all cylinders. The majority of people don't show symptoms of chronic illness (high blood pressure, fatigue, weight gain) until they're in their 40s. Fact.

Years of acid-forming foods, environmental pollution, and chemical invasion add up. Truth: Your cells have a natural life cycle, and every cell in your body will die at some point. Another truth: You can hasten said life cycle by chemically polluting your cells.

Top ten reasons to pay attention to your diet

A poor diet, which means consistently eating unhealthy foods, can set the stage for disease in your body. It's like issuing an invitation to a hungry vampire — you open the door to disease and it's going to come in. Check out these diseases that may be preventable with attention to diet and nutrition:

✔ Anemia

✔ Certain cancers (such as colon, bladder, and breast)

✔ Colds and flu virus

✔ Diabetes

✔ Gallstones

✔ Gout

✔ Heart disease (includes high blood pressure, cholesterol, and heart attack)

✔ Metabolic syndrome (a collection of symptoms, such as high blood pressure and a large midsection, that may herald more serious diseases, such as diabetes)

✔ Obesity

✔ Stroke

Shut the door on disease (and vampires) by eating a healthy, balanced diet full of vitamins and minerals. Proven fact: You can cut your risk of many diseases with proper nutrition.

I wish I could tell you exactly what symptom to look for, but I can't. Years of chronic acidity manifest differently in each of us. You have an individual fingerprint; likewise, your individual genes, or DNA, dictate your weakest link. Mine is skin; an acid-eating party results in an acne outbreak. You may have a nervous system weakness, with lethargy and irritability your only outward symptoms of an imbalanced pH. Chances are, you already know where your systemic weakest link lies.

Getting Started

Before you get started, I'd like to issue a word of warning to anyone with an existing disease or condition who hopes to cure it through diet. First, congrats to you for taking charge of your body, nutrition, and lifestyle. Now I have to add a caveat: Please talk to your doctor before you get started. Changes in diet can affect medical treatment and prescription regiments, and I don't want you to lose the benefit of any treatment or drug.

Staying the course

If excuses were worth money, I'd be a rich woman. It's human nature to rationalize bad decisions, so I'm not picking on anyone. I only encourage reflecting on why you stopped a healthy diet, exercise, or lifestyle. Was it too hard? Not fiscally feasible? No results?

The acid alkaline diet is a lifelong journey. You won't be done with it in a few months (hopefully). There are no complications in eating healthy, alkaline-forming foods for the rest of your life.

Giving yourself time to adjust

You're going to want to quit at some point. You may rationalize that you already feel better, it's too hard, or you just plain want to stop and go back to a more comfortable, let alone unhealthy, way of eating.

Give your body some time to get accustomed to the alkaline-forming foods. Many of them, like the cruciferous veggies, are full of fiber and can cause bloating and gas until you get accustomed to the extra fiber. But trust me, your colon will dance a jig when it realizes that these healthy foods are here to stay and that you've stopped filling it with chemicals and processed foods.

Chapter 2

You Are What You Eat

*U*nderstanding how to tell the difference between an *acidic* food and an *acid-forming* food is the cornerstone of the acid alkaline diet. If you have a question about a specific food choice, Chapter 11 is a good place to look. This chapter helps you understand what makes a food acid-forming or alkalinizing, and how to pair that knowledge with a nutritional balance.

The basis of implementing any diet, including this one, is centered on understanding your body's nutritional needs, and then learning how to incorporate the right food selections in your diet. Unless you enjoy carrying around papers telling you what you can and cannot eat on this diet, this knowledge will give you the power to start making better choices for your pH balance on your own.

 Step away from search engines if you're looking for reliable information on following an acid balanced diet — you'll find nothing but hoards of conflicting information on the web (and get incredibly frustrated in the process). The Internet is full of alkaline food lists, but many of them are very misleading.

Acidifying Foods Versus Acidic Foods

The problem, and the reason that the numerous acid alkaline food lists on the Internet are so confusing and contradictory, is that their creators probably don't grasp the difference between *acidic* and *acidifying*.

An *acidic* food, such as a lemon, references the food's pH, *not* how it impacts your body. An *acidifying* food, such as red meat, has an impact on your body, dropping your pH as it's processed by your digestive system.

Acidic foods are not always acidifying. After digestion, foods and beverages leave a residue in the digestive system, commonly referred to as an ash. The pH of this residue is what makes a food acidifying or alkalinizing — not it's pH before you eat it.

The following foods are highly acidic before digestion, but alkalize the body after digestion:

- ✔ Apple cider vinegar
- ✔ Lemons and lemon juice
- ✔ Limes and lime juice
- ✔ Oranges, tangerines, and grapefruit (just the fruits, not the juices which have concentrated sugar and are acid-forming)
- ✔ Tomatoes

Understanding the digestive process

The second a food or beverage enters your mouth, your body begins to digest it in two ways: chemically, through an enzyme release; and mechanically, through chewing. When you swallow, the food travels down your esophagus into your stomach, where both chemical and mechanical digestion continues.

Amazing acid container

Your stomach houses the most *acidic* substance in your body: *hydrochloric acid.* Also known as *gastric acid*, hydrochloric acid has a pH between 1 and 2, which means it's millions of times more acidic than plain water (pH 7.0). Food is broken down to smaller, more digestible parts using the mechanical churning of your stomach, gastric acid, and special digestive enzymes.

Hydrochloric acid is extremely caustic — it can cause burns to the skin. The stomach is lined with a special mucous membrane to protect it from digesting itself.

Entering your small intestine

As food leaves your stomach, it's pushed into the small intestine where the majority of nutrient absorption and true digestion occur. This is where your pH becomes affected, not in your stomach as some acid alkaline nay-sayers tout.

How long does digestion take?

From the moment you swallow to the moment you sit on the toilet, the digestive process can take up to 40 hours, give or take. After you swallow, food enters the stomach almost instantly. The stomach houses food for up to four hours, depending on the type of food. Typically, carbohydrates stay in your stomach for the briefest period, followed by proteins, with fats taking the longest to leave. Food can linger in the small intestine and colon (large intestine) for up to 36 hours. This lag time depends on how much fluid you drink, how healthy you are,

and whether you exercise (exercise increases blood flow, which can speed up digestion). This is why I can't tell you *exactly* when a food or beverage will impact your pH — it all depends on your digestive speed.

The exception to this rule involves fluids — which pass freely from your stomach to your small intestine unless they are barricaded by food. Have you ever had an alcoholic beverage on an empty stomach? Did it go "straight to your head"? It's because there is no food to slow the digestion.

People opposed to the acid alkaline diet — and there are a few — state that hydrochloric acid neutralizes all alkaline foods, therefore you cannot influence your pH through diet. This is only half true: Hydrochloric acid does break down food and alter the pH, but the remaining food residue in your small intestine is what influences your pH, not the gastric acid of your stomach.

At this point, other digestive organs (the liver and pancreas) join the party and release special enzymes that break down fat, carbohydrates, and protein in the small intestine. The combined effort breaks down the "food" (it's no longer recognizable as such) into tiny molecules. Finger-like projections in the small intestine absorb these molecules of water, minerals, vitamins, nutrients, and the ash from food digestion.

This is when the acidic or alkaline ash directly impacts your pH. Your body deals with each type of ash differently:

- **Acidic ash:** Your body releases alkaline buffers (usually calcium from your bones) to neutralize this ash.
- **Alkaline ash:** This type of ash typically doesn't start a reaction. Your body doesn't need to do anything special to alkaline ash because it has plenty of natural acids that routinely deal with alkaline substances.

Waxing from acid to alkaline

To understand how an acidic food can have an alkalizing effect, consider the humble lemon: A lemon sitting on a shelf has an acidic pH of around 4.0

(remember, 7.0 is neutral). It also contains minerals, which are alkalizing. When you eat a lemon, its citric acid is quickly broken down and neutralized in the powerful hydrochloric acid of your stomach. As the digested lemon enters your small intestine, it is broken down into tiny molecules for absorption. These remaining particles — the ash — consist of only alkalizing ash and minerals.

So lemons are an alkaline-forming food, even though they're acidic by nature.

Applying the 80/20 Rule

When you stick to a strict acid alkaline diet, 80 percent of your foods should be alkalinizing, with only 20 percent acid-forming. Apply this rule to every meal, beverage, and snack — basically *everything* you put in your mouth.

The 80/20 rule is a guideline for people wishing to cleanse their body and return to an alkaline state — it doesn't have to be a way of life. Many people survive happily on a 60/40 alkaline diet, meaning 60 percent of their foods are alkaline and 40 percent are acid-forming foods. Usually, this ratio is used to sustain good health — it won't correct years of acidity, but it helps you maintain a healthy balance moving forward.

So what's the right combination? Whatever works for you. This is not an exact science. The problem is that the majority of people currently live on an acid-forming diet composed of pasta, sweets, and caffeine. Mainstream society treats processed foods like one of the five main food groups — a daily visit to the drive-thru is not uncommon in many countries. Consider your lifestyle, activity level, and culinary capabilities as you decide what percent of your diet will become alkaline.

If you're an active type, you may benefit from a more alkaline diet because exercise breeds acid. If you're using the diet to improve your health or combat a disease process, more alkalinizing foods are always better.

Planning on 80 percent alkalinizing

Eating 80 percent alkalinizing foods isn't as challenging as it may first sound. Put away the scales and calculators, and use my easy way to keep the majority of your plate alkalinizing — just eyeball it and make food exchanges.

If you look at a plate from the typical standard American diet (SAD) you may see a couple acidifying starches (rolls, French fries), a red meat (hamburger, steak), and an acidifying beverage (beer, milk). A couple quick exchanges make this plate alkalinizing rather than acid-forming:

✔ Rather than buns and fries, choose yeast-free breads or wild rice

✔ Rather than red meat, choose white meat, seafood, or meat substitute

✔ Rather than milk or alcohol, choose water or sugar-free juice

It's very difficult to over-do it eating alkalinizing foods. If you fill up the majority of your plate with alkaline-forming foods, you will meet or exceed the 80/20 rule.

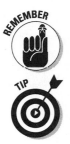

You can still enjoy your favorite acidifying foods every once in a while. If today's the day I'm going to enjoy a chocolate bar (acidifying), I make sure to drink plenty of water and eat an extra cup of vegetables throughout the day to combat the acids I form with the candy.

Understanding how to balance acidifying food with healthy alkalinizing choices allows you to seamlessly implement the acid alkaline diet into your life. To maximize the alkaline-forming foods on your plate consider the following:

✔ Create your snack or meal around a fruit or vegetable, not a meat or starch.

✔ Fill your plate with plant foods first, leaving little room for acid-forming meats and breads.

✔ Swap out acid-forming sides, such as dinner rolls, for an extra vegetable.

✔ Get creative preparing plant foods — they don't have to be boring. Chopped veggies with dip and grilled fruit can bring the fun back into eating healthy. (Check out the recipes in Part 4.)

✔ Think about what's on your plate — is the majority of your food natural and unaltered?

✔ Pay attention to hidden acids in dressings, condiments, and drinks. *Hidden acids* are sneaky little buggers that can be disguised as flavorings, spreads, sauces, dressings, and sweeteners. If you didn't make it yourself, skip the spreads and dressings, or request them on the side.

Limiting acids to 20 percent

Some foods are more or less acid forming in their various forms. Although all forms are acidic, some are worse than others. For example, although both eggs and milk are acid-forming foods, egg whites and no-fat milk have less impact on your pH.

If you fill your plate with healthy alkalinizing choices, you shouldn't have to work too hard to restrict your remaining acid-forming foods (unless you make a Scooby-Doo-style sandwich that goes to the ceiling). It's okay to have some acid-forming foods on your plate, as long as they're offset by alkaline-forming foods. Say you put a couple French fries on your dinner plate (you're only human after all). Combat the acid-forming potential of those fries with a bowl of salad or a cup of steamed broccoli. This may not create the ultimate alkalizing dinner plate, but it reduces the amount of acidic ash in your intestine during digestion.

When you plan your meals or build your plate, consider choosing the less acid-forming food. You can swap out red meat for chicken or pick an extra lean cut of beef rather than a fatty hamburger mix. Table 2-1 shows how to make better choices for your pH when selecting acid-forming foods.

Table 2-1	Choosing the Least Acidic Foods
Acidic Choice	*Less Acidic Choice*
Red meat or organ meat	Chicken, seafood
Whole egg	Egg white or egg substitute
White rice, white potatoes	Wild rice, sweet potatoes
Yeasted bread	Yeast-free bread
Yogurt	No-fat yogurt
Whole milk	Skim or no-fat milk
Sugar	Honey

Getting the Right Nutrients

You could eat nothing but spinach all day every day, and pat yourself on the back for eating such an alkalizing diet. However, you wouldn't be getting the nutrients your body needs to function properly, and your health would eventually decline. Ever hear people talk about eating a well-balanced diet? The term refers to the balance of nutrients, including vitamins and minerals, which can only be obtained from eating a variety of healthy foods.

If you don't eat a balanced diet, you won't reap the benefits of pH balance. Your body is always working hard in the background to correct dietary insufficiencies, but these corrections come at a cost to your overall health.

If you severely restrict any nutrient, your body tries to replace the deficit. Don't eat enough calcium? Your body steals it from your teeth and bones. Don't get enough protein? Your body breaks down muscle mass and steals the proteins. Balancing your diet is the only way to prevent your body from becoming a common criminal!

The nutrients you need to survive can be broken down into two main categories: the macronutrients and the micronutrients. As their name implies, the *macronutrients* are the ones you need the most of — the big guns in your diet. The *micronutrients* are the teeny tiny parts that make your body's functions work better.

Including lots of macronutrients

Macronutrients are the dietary heavy-hitters you need to survive. Each nutrient has a specific purpose within your body and is an important part of a balanced diet.

- ✔ **Carbohydrates** are the main energy source for your body.
- ✔ **Protein** builds and repairs every cell, including your skin and muscles.
- ✔ **Fat** protects your organs and helps you use vitamins A, D, E, and K.

All three macronutrients provide an energy source for your body. Carbohydrates are the foremost source of energy, followed by fat and protein.

If you don't ingest enough of a macronutrient, your body will find a way to replace deficits, but may acidify itself in the process. If you go on a fad, starvation-type diet, your body will break down and burn stored fats and proteins (your muscles) for the energy it needs to survive.

No carbs = no pH balance

If you decide to cut out carbohydrates (say you start a certain trendy diet that teaches you carbs are evil) your body eventually starts burning fat and protein instead of carbohydrates for energy. Just think — your body starts to burn the very same thing you're avoiding — animal protein and fat. It's just ironic that you're burning your own protein and fat! Plus, the byproduct of this switch is acid accumulation.

When you think about it, the nasty side effects associated with low-carb diets mirror the effects of acidification of your body. A low-carb dieter may experience some degree of:

- ✔ Lethargy
- ✔ Irritability
- ✔ Energy loss
- ✔ Memory problems
- ✔ Hunger
- ✔ Ketone release (byproduct of liver's attempt to create energy, *acidifies the blood*)

If you are a chronic low-carb dieter and want to start balancing your pH, you can resume balanced nutrition by slowly adding high-quality carbohydrates (fruits and vegetables) back into your diet. This may help you avoid gastrointestinal distress from the dietary shift including the side effects of bloating, gas, and constipation.

Fiber and water are not included in the official macronutrients, but they're also essential to your diet. Fiber acts as a broom to your colon, sweeping out extra cholesterol and gunk. Water is the bus to your waste — it transports acids out of your system and is essential for life. (I delve deeper into fiber in Chapter 12 and water in Chapter 6.)

The dietary recommendations for each macronutrient vary according to your gender, health, and age. Every decade or so, the recommendations are reviewed and updated by the World Health Organization (WHO) and the Food and Agriculture Organization (FAO) based on the needs and health of the general population. Table 2-2 shows the current average adult requirements for each macronutrient along with sources for each.

Table 2-2 Macronutrient Requirements for the Average Adult

Macronutrient	Recommendation	Sources
Carbohydrate	130 grams per day	Fruit, vegetables, grains, natural sugars
Protein	46 - 56 grams per day	Animal products, vegetables, seeds, nuts, legumes, soy
Fat	20 - 35 grams per day	Oils, dairy, fish, seeds, nuts, meat, poultry, dairy

United States Department of Agriculture. Dietary Reference Intakes: Macronutrients. National Agricultural Library.

Getting enough micronutrients

You can't see them with your naked eye, but tiny micronutrients are oh so good for you. Micronutrients include minerals and vitamins — those tiny elements in food necessary for survival.

These essential nutrients act in the background as catalysts, or the triggers that spark enzyme and chemical reactions throughout your body. These chemical reactions are involved in every living process including healing, growth, digestion, breathing — they even keep your heart beating.

Micronutrients have a key role in pH balance; many of the vitamins and minerals in certain foods are what makes them alkalinizing or acid-forming! It's not by coincidence that the majority of alkalinizing foods are plant foods, which are packed with vitamins and minerals.

The list of known vitamins and minerals is extensive; it would take an entire chapter just to cover these micronutrients in any depth, so I'm not going to try. The most important thing to know is that vitamins and minerals have a *symbiotic relationship* — they work interdependently and one is not more important than the other. Talk to your doctor if you are self-supplementing with specific vitamins and minerals — you may not be getting the mix right.

Filling Your Plate with Plants

Don't go munching on your gardenias (although they are edible). I'm talking about filling your plate with healthy plant foods including vegetables, fruits, seeds, nuts, and legumes — almost everything that grows from the earth.

If you force yourself to eat a plain salad with every meal — yawn — you won't reap the benefits of variety, and you will get bored. There are better ways to make sure you get plant foods on your plate and maintain variety in the process. For starters, if you're an iceberg-only lettuce-eater, it may be time to start experimenting with other greens including kale, watercress, and spinach.

Take baby steps and add one new vegetable per week. You don't want your system to go into shock at the dinner table — that never ends well.

If you're on a tight budget, purchasing seasonal fruits and vegetables and freezing or canning them is usually less expensive than paying over-the-top prices for fresh berries in winter. Or you can experiment growing your own produce. If you decide to plant an edible garden, take some advice from me: onions, peppers, tomatoes, cucumbers, strawberries, and zucchini are really hard to kill and produce a lot of fruit and vegetables to harvest.

Every plant has intrinsic vitamins and minerals, which vary from plant to plant. Spinach and kale are full of calcium, peppers contain vitamin C, and carrots have beta-carotene . . . get the idea? Keep it varied and aim for at least two cups of fruits and two cups of vegetables every day. You can build an entire meal around plant foods, which helps you adhere to alkalinizing food choices while maintaining a nutritionally balanced meal.

This list shows you how plant foods can take center stage for each meal:

- ✓ **Breakfast:** Fresh fruit, vegetable omelet, homemade almond granola
- ✓ **Lunch:** Salads, vegetable-based soups, grilled fruit
- ✓ **Dinner:** Steamed vegetables, tofu-based casseroles, legumes
- ✓ **Snacks:** Fruit or vegetable based smoothie, raw vegetables, toasted almonds

Although the majority of plant foods are naturally alkalinizing, a few form acid during digestion, so limit your intake of the following:

✔ **Fruits:** Blueberries, cranberries, plums, prunes, and raisins

✔ **Legumes:** Black beans, kidney beans, cashews, and peanuts

✔ **Vegetables:** Corn, olives, and white potatoes

Starchy vegetables, legumes, and sweet fruits are high on the *glycemic index,* which is a way of measuring the load of simple carbohydrates (sugar) in a food. It is believed that their high sugar content is acidifying during digestion. The other plant foods listed form an acidic ash during digestion, although they are still far less acidifying than animal proteins.

All Grains Are Not Created Equal

As a plant food, grains are an important source of fiber, carbohydrates, minerals, and vitamins. But they are not all created (or made) equally. Understanding how to select the best grains for your pH can save you a lot of frustration while you're trying to get it balanced.

Understanding whole grains

Whole grains are nothing more than edible seeds — the whole, intact seed is considered a whole grain. Each seed has three components:

✔ **Bran:** The outer layer

✔ **Endosperm:** The middle layer

✔ **Germ:** The inner core

Think about a kernel of popcorn. The tough outer skin is the bran, the inner starch includes the endosperm, and the teeny tiny seed at the center is the germ. Refining a grain removes all of the nutrients and fiber and strips it down to its starchy center part, the germ. The germ is nothing more than a simple carbohydrate, which breaks down easily into sugar during digestion.

Depending on their composition, some whole grains are acid-forming during digestion. Table 2-3 depicts acid-forming whole grains versus alkalinizing grains.

Table 2-3	Acidifying and Alkalinizing Grains
Acidifying Grain	*Alkalinizing Grain*
Wheat	Barley
White and brown rice	Wild rice
Rye	Oats
Corn meal	Quinoa
Buckwheat	Millet
White and wheat flour	Spelt or millet flour

Avoiding processed grains

Stripped of their protective coating, or bran, grains are considered processed or refined. Some processed grains are then *fortified,* or *enriched,* meaning that nutrients, such as fiber and the B and E vitamins, are artificially returned to the grain.

Processed grains are *always* acidifying. The beneficial fiber and pH balancing nutrients live in the bran and endosperm, which is removed during processing. All you're left with is a chewy morsel of germ, like white rice, that has absolutely no nutritional value and is full of empty calories.

Balancing grains

If you have that deer-in-the-headlights feeling when shopping for grains, don't worry, you're not alone. So many labels to read, so little time! Suffice it to say that any label reading *enriched*, *processed*, *milled,* or *fortified* does not enclose a natural product, and the food product inside will ultimately acidify you. (I offer a complete breakdown of acid-forming and alkalinizing foods in Chapter 11.)

Recommendations for grain consumption average around six servings per day, half of those being in the form of whole grains. But what constitutes a serving? You may be surprised. Think about the last plate of pasta you enjoyed at a restaurant. Chances are, you were given almost four times the recommended serving size of one ounce.

Yes, one measly ounce equals a serving of grains. This equates to:

- One slice of bread (not Texas gargantuan style — we're talking regular sliced bread)
- Half a cup of cooked rice
- Half a cup of cooked pasta
- A quarter of a deli-sized bagel
- Half a cup of cooked oats
- Half of a small English-style muffin

You don't need to break out a scale or measuring cups (although it may be beneficial to see how much pasta really fits in 1/2 cup) to make sure you aren't overdoing it with grains. One ounce of a grain food is about the size of half a baseball or about half the size of your closed fist.

Limiting the Meats You Eat

Almost every type of animal flesh has a negative impact on your pH. However, there are degrees of acidification — with red meats being on the really acidifying end of the spectrum and fish and poultry on the other. For some people, giving up (or reducing) meat may be the hardest part of adhering to the acid alkaline diet.

A *serving* of meat is three ounces — about the size of a deck of cards.

Research shows that taking small steps, making exchanges here and there, helps you adhere to permanent dietary and lifestyle changes.

Ditching the reds

Red meat comes from both livestock and wild animals. These meats have the biggest impact on your pH and are extremely acid-forming in your body.

The red meats include:

- Beef (and veal)
- Bison
- Duck and goose
- Goat
- Lamb (and mutton)

- ✔ Pork
- ✔ Rabbit

Red meat consumption is directly linked to several different types of cancer (including breast and colon cancer), high blood pressure, and heart disease. Research shows that each additional serving of red meat correlates with an increased risk of death from disease.

I can't tell you to quit eating red meat (I'm not trying to create an army of vegans, after all). What I am saying is that red meat, no matter how little you eat, directly impacts your pH and leaves an acidic ash in your small intestine. If you're ready to give up the red meats, start by swapping out a serving of red meat for a serving of white meat, seafood, or a plant protein.

If you must eat red meat, pay attention to meat quality, serving size, and avoid processed meat (luncheon meat, hot dogs, and other unnatural creations) like the plague. Always choose quality red meat, not the ground up who-knows-what-it-is meat. Lean cuts have very little marbling (the white veining is actually stores of saturated fat) and usually hide under the guise of flank, eye of round, and sirloin.

If you eat meat, don't overdo. Step away from the 12-ounce rib-eye special — it provides four servings of red meat in one sitting!

The great protein debate

By far, the number one question posed by friends after they knew I'd dropped meat from my diet was, "Where do you get your iron and protein?" Why are we so protein crazed? Yes, it is the building block of all cells in your body. Yes, it helps you heal and builds and repairs muscle tissue, but meat isn't the only source of protein. Legumes, nuts, seeds, seafood, and plants provide protein without the side dish of saturated fat found in red meat.

Red meat lovers may try to convince you that animal meats are the only complete source of

- ✔ Fatty acids
- ✔ Conjugated linoleic acid (CLA) — an antioxidant
- ✔ Iron and zinc
- ✔ Protein (it contains *all of the essential amino acids*, or building blocks of protein, for health)

All of these nutrients are found in plant foods. Nuts provide fatty acids, plant-based oils are a source of CLA, iron and zinc are abundant in leafy green vegetables and beans, and tofu is a complete protein source, just like red meat.

Picking poultry

Poultry and seafood are by far the best animal protein choices for your pH. If you adhere to the proper serving size and don't overdo it with frequency, the impact on your pH can be negligible. But don't make the common mistake of thinking all poultry is in the green zone — that fast-food drive-thru poultry doesn't really count (I'm not even sure some of it is chicken).

Have you noticed the wall of poultry selections available at the grocery store? You have your basic whole bird, and about 30 other selections ranging from pre-seasoned pieces to neat little rows of drumsticks. Skip the pre-seasoned pieces and birds, unless you know exactly what's in that rub. Personally, I like the breast tenderloins. Each piece is equal to about a serving of meat and they're skinless.

Dark meat? White meat? I say whatever floats your boat. Just be advised that dark meat has slightly more fat than white meat, which creates more acid ash during digestion.

Selecting seafood

Quality seafood selections can play a large role in your acid alkaline diet. Although all seafood is animal food, enjoying a three-ounce serving of seafood may not substantially impact your pH. Coldwater fish, such as wild-caught salmon, provide a healthy dose of *omega 3-fatty acids* — the fats that help protect against heart disease and stroke.

If you're currently ill, pregnant, or nursing, talk to your doctor before eating seafood, and avoid all raw seafood including certain types of sushi and clams or oysters on the half shell.

Oysters are an excellent source of vitamins and minerals including calcium, which is a potent alkaline source (they're also an aphrodisiac, but I'm not sure how that impacts your pH).

Mussels and shellfish (including shrimp, lobster, and scallops) are slightly acidifying. When you eat shellfish, make sure to keep an eye on serving sizes and don't exceed three ounces per meal (or five ounces per day).

Meeting the other white meats — soy and whey

Plant proteins provide a healthy alternative to animal meat. The "other white meats," including tofu and tempeh, come in a variety of forms that can easily replace almost any red meat or poultry in a recipe. Plus, since they are not derived of animal flesh, plant proteins form an alkaline ash during digestion.

Be careful when you shop for meat replacements — some of the current faux meat choices contain wheat protein (seitan), which is an acid-forming food.

Tofu

Made from soybean curds and water, tofu is a cholesterol-free, low-fat food. Each ½ cup tofu serving contains about ten grams of protein, which beats both eggs and cow milk gram for gram. This soy product is also an excellent source of calcium, providing between 100 and 200 milligrams of calcium per serving (depending on the brand and type).

Tofu comes in two main forms, each good for different uses:

- ✔ **Firm** or **extra-firm** is best for grilling, baking, and stir-frying.
- ✔ **Silken** works well for dressings, desserts, and smoothies.

Tofu tastes best when marinated or heavily seasoned (basically because it has no taste of its own). The next time you make a chili or stew, consider throwing in a few cubes of this alkalinizing protein.

Tempeh

Tempeh is also born of soybeans, but includes the entire bean and is fermented as opposed to curdled.

Tempeh has a distinct taste and texture, which can be dampened with boiling or braising prior to preparation. It tastes a little nutty (I don't mean crazy, I mean like actual nuts) and has a coarser texture than firm tofu. You can find tempeh in the refrigerated produce section at the store in many different shapes and sizes. (My store has tempeh "sausage" and tempeh "hot dogs.")

Whey

Although it is not a meat, whey is a good source of protein. Whey protein is one of the two milk proteins (casein is the other).

So what's up with the soy controversy?

Eat it. Don't eat it. Eat it. If your head's spinning based on the conflicting stories of soy's health benefits, you're not alone. Here are the facts posed by numerous studies:

✔ Soy products have minimal impact on cholesterol levels. (You can reduce your cholesterol by eating less fatty meat; there's no magic ingredient in the soy.)

✔ Soy isoflavone supplements are not recommended for anyone — eat it natural or not at all.

✔ Soy contains a chemical, phytoestrogen, which skeptics associate with the estrogen hormone in women. However, studies conclude that there isn't enough phytoestrogen in soy to benefit menopausal symptoms — in other words, the little bit of phytoestrogen in soy is insignificant.

✔ Soy is a not a miracle cure for people with high blood pressure, cancer, or other disease.

Although some animal studies have connected certain forms of soy, such as soy flour, with an increased cancer risk, this might be because they were feeding the poor little creatures mounds of the stuff, more than you or I would ever sit down and eat.

Whey protein isolate is a highly refined protein powder — it has been through multiple processes to skim off excess fat and milk sugars, resulting in a 99 percent pure protein product (although this may vary by manufacturer) that has very little fat or carbohydrates. Whey isolate is mostly lactose-free and is a gluten-free food.

You can add whey protein isolate powder to smoothies or enjoyed plain mixed with water.

Chapter 3

Detecting Acids in Your Body

. . . .

In This Chapter

▶ Recognizing signs of acidity

▶ Understanding body systems

▶ Discovering the most common effects of imbalance

▶ Observing systematic consequences

. . . .

*S*igns and symptoms are the outward indications that something is amiss in your body. The symptoms of pH imbalance are elusive. Indeed, it would be much easier if you developed huge purple triangles on your skin when your pH was out of whack — but that's not the case. Because each person has a different genetic make-up, my outward symptoms may not be the same as yours. Therefore, the list of pH imbalance symptoms in this chapter is quite extensive, but not all-inclusive.

You are the expert here — only you know when something in your body is not working as it should.

Your body is composed of a network of systems (12 to be exact) that work together to sustain health. These 12 systems include all of the bones, muscles, and major organs in your body. You may think this chapter doesn't pertain to you — but only through learning about your body can you understand what it's trying to tell you.

Recognizing Imbalance in Your Body's Systems

If you're an intuitive person, you may not need all the gadgets and pH test kits that I tell you about in Chapter 4 to recognize a pH imbalance. (Of course, they can be very helpful if you're at all like me and like instructions to boil an egg). Many practitioners of the acid alkaline diet say that you can feel the shift in your pH just by tuning into your body.

Many symptoms of pH imbalance reflect the system or systems impacted by acid overload. The easiest way to recognize this imbalance is by understanding what each system is meant to do when you are in a state of perfect health. Some early warning signs of a pH shift into acidic territory may include:

- ✔ **Digestive system:** Gastrointestinal problems — irregular bowels and bloating
- ✔ **Endocrine system:** Low energy levels
- ✔ **Integumentary system:** Skin problems — sudden breakouts and dryness
- ✔ **Nervous system:** Personality/memory changes — agitation and poor recall

My outward symptoms of acidity may not be the same as yours. I talk about keeping a journal in Chapter 4, which may help you identify your personal symptoms stemming from an acidic lifestyle and diet.

Do you recall your last fast food binge? Mine was last summer, as we celebrated the end of our children's baseball season. We gorged on burgers, fries, and milkshakes. Exactly two hours later, I felt fatigued, bloated, and had a nasty case of heartburn. It took about two hours for the fats and proteins from our meal to acidify my body. (So that's instant gratification of a sort!)

I am not a doctor, nor do I play one on television. Anytime you find a concerning symptom or something is not working right in your body, consult with your medical professional. Don't use this chapter to self-diagnose problems. It is intended as a reference — so you can learn more about common symptoms of acidity and how it can impact different parts of your body.

The nervous system

Including your brain, spinal cord, and a delicate web of nerves throughout your body, your nervous system allows you to interact with the environment. Do you smell coffee brewing? Hear a phone ringing? Your nervous system is constantly working in the background to catalogue these stimuli, and help your body respond (or ignore) them.

Your nervous system controls more than just your five senses, it also commands your emotional responses and cognitive functions. If you feel weepy or can't focus on the task at hand, your nervous system may be suffering from an imbalanced pH.

Symptoms of acid toxicity acting on your nervous system may include:

- ✔ Cold feet and hands
- ✔ Difficulty concentrating
- ✔ Feeling cold or chilly frequently in a warm room
- ✔ Headaches
- ✔ Irritability
- ✔ Loss of motivation
- ✔ Memory changes
- ✔ Sadness

The cardiovascular system

Your body contains a virtual roadmap of veins, arteries, and capillaries that circulate blood and nutrients throughout your body. Every single organ in your body is affected by the health of your cardiovascular system.

The human heart is nothing more than a pump — one side pushes blood and nutrients throughout your body, while the other side receives the exhausted blood (including cellular waste) for recycling. Chronic acid intake can lead to an *inflammatory response* (swelling of the tissues), which makes your cardiovascular system work harder to pump nutrients.

When your cardiovascular system is under acid attack you can suffer:

- ✔ Irregular heart beats
- ✔ High blood pressure
- ✔ Fast heart rate at rest

No *cardiologist* (heart doctor) will attribute your irregular heartbeat or cardiovascular problems completely to acidity and nor should you. Talk to your doctor right away if you are suffering any of these symptoms, as there can be other, more serious underlying causes that require medical treatment.

The same goes for the alkaline lifestyle extremists who claim that an acidic diet will lead to a heart attack. I won't dispute that the acidity can help set the stage for heart disease — but it's probably not the main focus when someone is suffering from a serious cardiovascular disease.

Checking your pulse

How do you know if your heart rate is irregular? Some people can feel their heart beating abnormally. Other people live with a chronically irregular heartbeat detected by checking a pulse or getting an *echocardiogram* (ECG), which is a representation of your heart's electrical activity on paper. If the irregularity is sporadic (intermittent or not chronic), the errant beats are called palpitations. Many factors impact your heart rate and could lead to palpitations including:

✔ Caffeine intake

✔ Sleeplessness

✔ Dietary insufficiencies (especially electrolytes and minerals)

✔ Exercise and activity level

✔ Hydration — when you're dehydrated, your heart beats faster to circulate what little fluid you have

✔ Smoking or tobacco use

✔ Recreational drug use

The easiest place to check your pulse is on the inside of your wrist.

1 Using the first two fingers of your dominant hand, gently place your fingertips on the inside of your other wrist, in a straight line with your thumb.

2 Exert a little pressure. You should feel a steady beat. If you cannot feel anything, slightly reposition your fingertips or press a little harder. If you press too hard, you can block the artery!

   If you still can't find anything, take my word for it — you have a pulse, you just can't feel it.

3 Once you feel a steady beat (pulse), take a look at the clock. Count the beats for one full minute, for 30 seconds (and multiply the result by 2), or for 15 seconds (and multiply the result by 4).

The average heart rate ranges 60 to 100 beats per minute.

The skeletal and muscular systems

Your skeletal and muscular systems are the only things stopping you from being a blob on the sidewalk. These systems provide the framework for your body, as well as energy and strength. That's the good news. The bad news is that these systems are easily influenced by your pH. Your bones and muscles need the alkaline environment provided by their innate minerals, such as calcium.

When the body is under an acid attack, it turns to your skeletal and muscular systems for a quick supply of *alkaline buffers* (minerals, such as calcium, that reverse an acidic pH) and steals what is necessary to bring the pH back up to an alkaline state. The resulting alkaline deficit can lead to:

- Cavities in your teeth
- Brittle bones (osteoporosis)
- Decreased energy, strength, and endurance
- Joint pain
- Fatigue
- Muscular wasting (unhealthy thin appearance)

The digestive system

The digestive system is the human equivalent to a car's gas tank. Including the digestive organs of the stomach, intestines, liver, gallbladder, and even the pancreas, this system is responsible for breaking down and absorbing nutrients from food and turning them into energy.

Your digestion is the first system impacted by an acidic diet, which is why you may feel these symptoms sooner than symptoms affecting other systems. Signs that your digestive system is affected by imbalanced pH may include:

- Bowel movement irregularities (constipation, diarrhea)
- Heartburn
- Gas and bloating
- Cramps

The integumentary system

Integument is a fancy name for your skin and associated structures (hair, nails, the fat underneath the skin). As the largest organ, your skin is your frontline barrier to disease and injury (just imagine walking around without skin to hold everything in — yuck!).

The outermost layer of your skin is slightly acidic, which works as an extra layer of protection to kill germs. Underneath that *acid mantle,* the layers of your skin have a delicate pH balance.

If you feed your body acidic foods, it flushes excess acid out through your skin. When acidity builds up in this system you may notice:

- Acne (especially acne vulgaris, which is inflammatory)
- Dry, peeling skin and eczema
- Sores at the corners of the mouth
- Weak, brittle nails
- Hair loss
- Yeast overgrowth (rashes, especially in rolls of skin)

The endocrine and reproductive systems

The endocrine system is composed of hormones and glands; these glands release hormones into your blood and lymph tissue that regulate functions in your body. If you're thinking about skipping to the next section, read this first: Your glands include your sexuality and reproductive system — and the testicles (men) and ovaries (women) can be impacted by acidity.

Your thyroid gland is part of the endocrine system. It releases hormones that help regulate your *metabolism* (how fast your body makes and uses energy). A chronically acidic diet and lifestyle can impair your metabolic rate, which in turn affects your energy production and fat burning capability — do you see a vicious cycle starting here? An acidic life can lead to acid build-up in fats, which can lead to an impaired metabolism, which leads to obesity.

Although they are elusive and harder to pin to acidic dietary choices, symptoms of acid build-up affecting the reproductive system can lead to:

- Low sperm count (in men)
- Acidic cervical mucous (in women, the acids act as a spermicide and can thwart fertility)
- Recurrent yeast infections
- Irregular menses (in women)

Impacts on the endocrine system can cause:

- Fatigue and lethargy
- Agitation and panic attacks
- Poor metabolism
- Obesity
- Diabetes Type II

Combating the yeastie beasties

Yeast is a fungus that rapidly divides and thrives on sugar. A certain type of yeast, *Candida albicans*, is the culprit for recurrent vaginal and oral yeast infections. This little fungus can invade your entire body if left unchecked (or if you have an unhealthy immune system).

Yeast consumption, in any form, is highly discouraged on the acid alkaline diet. These little yeastie beasties are already present all over your body — they live in your mouth, on your skin, and even colonize your intestines. Normally, your immune system keeps them in check with the help of good bacteria known as probiotics. However, if you are sick, damage your good bacteria (like when you take antibiotics), or when you overconsume them (in breads, pastries, canned goods), the yeast throw a party and start to multiply uncontrollably causing the burning, itching, and white overgrowth associated with oral and vaginal yeast infections.

But that's not all the yeast do — they also whisper to your cells, begging for more sugar. In response, you get a wicked sugar craving and feed the beast. Your pH drops, and a viscous cycle begins.

Want to break the cycle? Consider starving the yeast. If the yeastie beasties don't get food, they are unable to multiply and overgrow (again, unless you have an underlying disease process). They also hate garlic, which is known to have anti-fungal properties. This is one reason you'll see a lot of garlic in my recipe chapters — I love this delicious fungus-fighter!

The pulmonary system

Also known as the *respiratory system*, this system includes all the organs essential to the exchange of gases — breathing, in other words.

Secondary only to your digestive system, this system is bombarded with acids all day. The structures impacted by excess acids in this system include your nose, trachea, bronchi, and lungs. Pulmonary symptoms of acid build-up may include:

- ✔ Chronic cough
- ✔ Chronic sinus problems
- ✔ Post-nasal drip
- ✔ Excess mucous
- ✔ Rapid breathing

Your body will do whatever is necessary to regain pH balance — sometimes to your detriment. This is why the majority of acidic pulmonary symptoms are *chronic*, which means you experience them over long periods of time.

If you've ever witnessed a small child throwing a tantrum and holding their breath, you probably saw the following collapse of said child. When you hold your breath, you're holding in acids usually dispelled through exhalation. Your blood keeps on pumping to your lungs, bringing a fresh batch of acid with each heartbeat. It doesn't take long for your pH to drop and become acidic. Your brain then goes on red alert and hits your reboot button — shutting down all systems (making you pass out). This allows your breathing to return to regular and naturally corrects the pH imbalance.

The immune and lymphatic systems

Your immune system is your personal army — it prevents all would-be invading organisms, both foreign and domestic, from taking over and damaging your body. *Foreign organisms* include things such as a virus that's getting spread around the office, whereas *domestic organisms* include the fungus and bacteria that live within you — yeast, for example.

The immune system works hand-in-hand with your lymphatic system, which contains lymph nodes and vessels that collect and remove dead or diseased cells from your body.

That little paper cut on your finger? It doesn't become infected because your immune system is working to heal it the second you slice it, and your lymphatic system is wicking away the dead cells.

When your immune system isn't well, you aren't well. Signs of acid toxicity affecting your immune and lymphatic systems may include:

- Chronic sneezing and allergies
- Easily catching colds
- Skin eruptions and slow healing
- Low-grade fever (99.1)
- Fatigue
- Generalized aches and pains

The urinary system

The urinary system is one of your major *excretory* (waste ejecting) systems. It includes the kidneys, ureters, bladder, and urethra. Your kidneys work as giant filters, removing waste, acid, and other toxins from your body via urine. They are also the last stop for acids in your body.

The kidneys are constantly working to balance pH by regulating *bicarbonate*, a potent alkaline substance in your body. When your kidneys become overworked from chronic acidity you may notice:

- ✔ Urinary tract infections
- ✔ Kidney stones (compilation of acids and minerals)
- ✔ Disease and inflammation of the kidneys

Brewing Disease

"*The diseases which destroy a man are no less natural than the instincts which preserve him.*" Yeah, I wish I said that, but actually an American poet, George Santayana (1863–1952) gets the credit line. If you want the 21st century version, it would read something like, "You are what you eat" or "You reap what you sow," although those are far less poetic.

The acid alkaline diet has two main purposes:

- ✔ Reduce your body's work compensating for poor pH choices
- ✔ Remove cellular waste from years of acidifying intake

When either of these fail to happen, your body goes into compensation mode, in which your systems struggle to maintain a slightly alkaline pH — totally without your help. This is not the optimal arrangement, because your body will do anything to preserve your slightly alkaline state. The next few sections illustrate exactly what can happen when you allow acidity to build up and make your body do the pH balancing act.

Altering years of chronic acidity takes time. These chronic diseases did not develop overnight — they slowly infiltrated your body. Why do you think the majority of people don't show signs of chronic disease until they are in their 40s? The constant bombardment of acidic foods, beverages, and lifestyles slowly wear down your body until you have no disease-fighting reserve left.

I can't predict where or how your manifestation of chronic acidity will show. If you're genetically programmed to have a weaker gastrointestinal system than others, it may show in the form of chronic heartburn or gas. If your weakness lies with your skin, years of acidity may make in an appearance in the form of frequent blemishes.

Asthma

Right off the bat, let me exclude childhood asthma from this list. Unlike *adult-onset asthma* (people who never had asthma before who suddenly have it or its cousin, reactive airway disease), childhood asthma is a disease of the upper airways caused by an inappropriate response to *allergens* (substances that cause an allergic reaction). I'm not encouraging an alkaline-forming diet for children — this book is geared for the adult.

In the absence of any former (childhood) disease, when an adults develops asthma it's due to an overcompensation of the body or an inappropriately severe response to a simple allergen. In the perfectly healthy individual, a little pollen in the lungs shouldn't cause the coughing and wheezing characteristic of an asthma attack. Chronic exposure to allergens such as smoke, mold, and dust, as well as an acidic environment may contribute to the disease.

When your body is acidic, your lungs can pay the price with a chronic cough, frequent upper respiratory illnesses, and the bronchial spasms of asthma (or reactive airway disease).

Diabetes

Again, I am *not* talking about juvenile or childhood cases of diabetes. In later stages of life, some adults develop type II diabetes (which used to be called adult onset diabetes) as a result of decreasing or ineffective insulin production. *Insulin* is the hormone that neutralizes high levels of sugar in the blood.

Your pancreas is working hard to keep your blood sugar stable — even as you read this. Like anything else in your body, your pancreas can get tired from being chronically overworked. The Standard American Diet is a roller coaster of simple and complex sugars, which make your pancreas work overtime expelling insulin to maintain a stable blood sugar.

When you have a soft drink, your pancreas releases insulin. If it weren't for insulin, the sugar content in your blood would keep rising and eventually put you into a coma. Remember: Sugar is acid-forming; your body will enter a coma to stop all non-essential processes while it tries hard to correct the blood sugar and reset your pH (but it will fail without medical intervention).

Heart disease

Heart disease, if not hereditary, can become a secondary or tertiary effect of an acidic lifestyle. An acidic diet contains foods (fats and sugars) that may lead to obesity, high cholesterol, diabetes, and inflammation, all of which are known to set the stage for cardiovascular disease.

When your arteries fill with *plaque*, a substance that attaches itself to the inner arterial wall and inhibits blood supply, your arteries become narrow, which can lead to high blood pressure, coronary artery disease, and blood clotting. If blood clots travel to your brain, you have a stroke; if they get lodged in the arteries feeding your heart, you have a heart attack.

 A pH balanced diet cannot cure heart disease. What it can do is help reduce your risk factors for developing heart disease. I can't say, "poof" and make the dead tree branch that just caved my roof in disappear, but I could've trimmed the tree last year and removed the dead branches. It's easier to prevent heart disease than it is to fix it once it occurs.

Alzheimer's

There is currently no scientific proof that any diet can prevent or stop Alzheimer's disease. However, an acid alkaline diet encourages a combination of natural plant foods with healthy proteins, and the plaques found in the brains of Alzheimer's patients are a tangled mix of unhealthy proteins (forming neuritic and senile plaques).

 If you're caring for a loved one with Alzheimer's, you already know that mealtime can be challenging. Many healthy alkalinizing foods are well tolerated by the advanced Alzheimer's patient, including:

- ✔ Steamed vegetables
- ✔ Soft, sliced fruits
- ✔ Protein shakes

Arthritis

There are many different types of *arthritis* (inflammation of the joints), some of which cannot be cured with dietary or lifestyle changes (juvenile, or childhood arthritis for instance).

Caregivers and mealtime: A potentially painful mix

If you're providing care for a loved one, mealtimes can be a painful affair. Regardless of whether he suffers cancer, she has dementia, or both mom and dad have Alzheimer's, all the diseases seem to make your loved one abhor mealtime and getting nutrients. Try these methods to decrease mealtime frustration, for both you and your loved one:

✔ Try not to rush meals.

✔ Turn off the television, radio, and other distractions.

✔ Don't offer a buffet of food — the large spread is overwhelming and can result in a bout of agitation.

✔ Add one food at a time (don't offer a plate filled with a variety of foods).

✔ Stick to culinary favorites (if dad likes mac'n'cheese, make it).

✔ Offer frequent, small meals as opposed to three giant ones.

✔ Pack each meal with nutrition if your loved one needs to gain weight (add protein powder to drinks, mashed potatoes, or soup).

Certain types of arthritis (osteoarthritis, degenerative arthritis) may respond to the dietary and lifestyle changes encouraged by the acid alkaline diet. Simple carbohydrates, animal products, and fatty foods, all of which are limited on a pH balanced diet, are known to provoke arthritis pain and increase inflammation. On the other hand, pH-balancing foods such as fruits, vegetables, cold-water fish, and seeds are encouraged for arthritis sufferers, because their vitamins and minerals can help decrease inflammation.

TECHNICAL STUFF

Gout is a form of arthritis provoked by an intake of red meats, alcohol, and seafood. Tiny crystals of uric acid lodge in the joint space and cause significant pain, swelling, and redness in the joint.

TIP

Talk to your doctor about dietary changes while on prescription medication for arthritis. Many people can benefit from a mainly alkalinizing diet, which is a natural low-fat source of dietary fiber, vitamins (such as vitamin E), and minerals.

Osteoporosis

Fact: To correct a pH drop into acidity, your body steals calcium, a potent alkalinizing source, from your bones. Over time, this theft decreases bone density, making bones brittle and easily prone to fractures. This loss of bone density is called *osteoporosis*.

Many factors increase your risk for osteoporosis including:

✔ Dietary deficiencies of calcium or vitamin D

✔ Genes — family history of the disease

✔ Hormone replacement use

✔ Smoking

✔ Alcohol consumption

Cancer

As much as I'd love to, I can't say a diet will cure cancer. However, a diet rich in plant foods and low in saturated fats and sugar may decrease your risk of cancer or cancer recurrence. Researchers are also finding that cancer cells thrive on sugar, which is strictly limited on the acid alkaline diet.

Scientific studies have yet to isolate which phytochemicals contribute to the cancer-fighting property of an alkaline-based diet. A *phytochemical* is a compound found in raw plant foods that keeps the plants healthy and vibrantly colorful while they are living. The bright green coloring of spinach comes from a phytochemical called chlorophyll and the vivid orange of pumpkins comes from carotenoids.

Table 3-1 lists the numerous phytochemicals known to reduce your risk of chronic disease, such as cancer.

Table 3-1	Disease-Fighting Phytochemicals
Phytochemical	*Source*
Carotenoids	Pumpkin, carrots
Chlorophyll	Spinach, parsley
Curcumin	Turmeric
Flavonoids	Tea, chocolate
Soy Isoflavones	Soybeans
Lignans	Seeds, nuts
Phytosterols	Nuts, legumes
Resveratrol	Grapes, red wine

Observing Acidosis

As you read this, your body may be compensating for acidity. Unless you have uncomfortable symptoms, you may be completely unaware of it — but it's happening, regardless.

As a young man or woman, your body continues to grow and develop. It has plenty of reserve left to fight off the effects of acidity. As you age, that reserve decreases. This is when the signs and symptoms of an acid-forming lifestyle start to surface — when your body is too busy sustaining life to worry about cleaning house and removing acidic build-up. The signs could start to rear their ugly head in your 30s or 40s — it's different for individuals based on your genetic make up.

Identifying premature aging

The fountain of youth is real — it lives within you. Premature (early) aging occurs when the body is abused and cannot continue to fight both the constant battle of bad lifestyle choices and environmental attacks. It's so busy trying to compensate for what you did (or didn't do) today, that it doesn't have any reserves left to fix prior waste build-up.

Why the wrinkles?

Fine lines, crow's feet, parenthesis, crinkles, creases, or deep furrows — most people hate them no matter what they're called. Unless you're an infant, skin wrinkles are an outward sign of aging (and wisdom).

Wrinkles have five main causes:

- Unprotected sun exposure
- Heredity
- Skin type (the darker the pigment the better)
- Environment (smoking, pollution)
- Diet and hydration

Wrinkles are the effect of tired skin. As you age, years of dietary and environmental abuse start to show in the form of spots and wrinkles. Although today's technological cosmetic advances (plastic surgery, lasers, and creams) can help reverse some of the signs of aging, you can reduce a few risk factors on your own:

- Never sit in the sun unprotected.
- Stop smoking or using tobacco.
- Eat a diet rich in antioxidants (such as plant foods).
- Keep yourself hydrated by drinking plenty of water and avoiding dehydrating beverages, such as those with caffeine or alcohol.

Just imagine what would happen if you stopped taking your garbage out. It would build up in your kitchen and eventually spill over into your entire home. The festering garbage would soon attract rodents, insects, and bacteria. It wouldn't take too long for your house to be condemned and for the entire structure to become uninhabitable. When it comes to your bodily wastes, you are the house — when you feed your body acids, you damage the entire structure and invite parasites such as disease and illness.

Although they count, wrinkles and skin damage are not the only warning signs of premature aging. When you begin to age, each body system is impacted with a:

- ✔ Loss of lean muscle tone (weight gain)
- ✔ Loss of subcutaneous fats (wrinkles and feeling chilled)
- ✔ Loss of skin elasticity (wrinkles)
- ✔ Slowing metabolism (weight gain)
- ✔ Decreased visual acuity (eyesight changes)
- ✔ Decreased immune function
- ✔ Decreased cardiovascular function (decreased blood supply to the skin and organs)

Premature aging is accelerated with poor dietary and lifestyle choices. It's argued that an acid-forming lifestyle bathes your *DNA* (the little cells and genes that are your blueprint) in waste, which speeds up cellular mutations and leads to an aging body.

The wastes are called *free radicals* — an accumulation of trash from cellular processes (breathing, eating, making energy). You can't stop free radicals from forming in your body. You can help your body remove the free radicals by eating an alkaline-based diet rich in plant foods. Plant foods contain various nutrients, such as vitamins, that act as *antioxidants*. Concentrated in vitamins A, C, and E, antioxidants are your personal garbage men — they float through your body and neutralize all of the free radicals.

Acquiring obesity

When your calorie intake exceeds your body's needs, the excess calories are stored as fat. This fat contains acid, and your body quickly tucks it away to protect vital organs. Worse yet, your body is smart enough to know this, so it goes one step further and decreases the blood supply to the fat, stopping the acids from re-entering circulation.

What does this mean to you? You now have a reservoir of fat that is stowed away, difficult to reach, and genetically biased. The location of your fat depot is genetically determined, however women tend to store these acids on their hips, buttocks, and thighs, whereas men store it on their waist.

If you have been struggling with weight loss, even after proper diet and exercise, you may actually be struggling with acidity. Chapter 6 goes into more detail about exercise, weight loss, and your pH.

Chapter 4

Your Acid Alkaline Toolkit

In This Chapter

▶ Testing your pH

▶ Keeping a descriptive journals

▶ Monitoring results

▶ Watching for changes

*U*nless you're my identical twin, your pH won't respond to anything the exact same way as mine. Many publications about the pH diet focus on lists telling you what to and not to eat. And although I provide rough guidelines (and a list in Chapter 11), the real focus of this book — and a pH balanced diet — is to illustrate how nutrition and lifestyle affect you.

Individual diet preferences and tolerances may exclude some items on standardized food lists. By mastering the basics of pH testing, you can overcome a slavish reliance on a food list, discover what impacts your personal pH, and make the subtle changes you need to keep your body functioning at its best.

This chapter gives you step-by-step instructions on how to test the pH of urine, saliva, and even foods and beverages (but remember, the pre-digestive pH of a food does not necessarily indicate its effects on your body). Pull out your lab coat . . . you're about to have some fun!

Testing Your pH

Testing your pH at home is the easiest way to determine your pH balance. You can do this using a type of litmus paper and body fluids (urine or saliva). *Litmus paper* is a chemically treated paper that reflects the pH of the liquid you dip it in.

Wading through the cobwebs in my brain, I recall using litmus paper in high school chemistry, but it was very basic (no pun intended). That paper turned red in acidic solutions and blue in alkaline solutions. It looked and felt much like a coffee filter (actually, some people make their own litmus strips at home using coffee filters and red cabbage . . . but that's another story).

You can purchase litmus paper in a small roll or in single use strips. On average, you get about 50 feet on a roll or 100 single use strips in one package. (The roll is far more economical. Since you use three-inch pieces for each test, you get about 200 tests out of the roll.) You can find this pH testing paper in health food stores or online.

Many different brand names and types of pH test strips are available, ranging in price from about 10 to 22 U.S. dollars — depending on how fancy you want them. Some test kits come with a CD-ROM instructional, sample diets, and even sample cups for testing specimen collection.

Unless you want to spend more money than you have to, all you really need is a pH testing kit that includes

✔ Testing paper or strips

✔ Color match guide

✔ Instructions

The paper colors vary — some turn red, yellow, or even a shade of tan to reflect acidity. This is why the strips come with a color match guide, which is a sheet of paper either in the bottle or on the side of the packaging. The colors equate to a pH reading that usually ranges from 5 to 9 on the linear pH scale.

Although a pH of 6 may not sound much worse than a pH of 7, the scale is exponential. Each 1-point move towards acidity or alkalinity represents a power of ten. If my pH tests at 6 and yours tests at 7, I'm 10 times more acidic than you. Similarly, if my pH is 5 and yours is 7, I'm 100 times more acidic than you (and so forth and so on). For the most accurate readings, be sure to buy strips that measure pH at least to the tenths (6, 6.5, 7, 7.5) and not just whole numbers (6,7,8).

Read the packaging on your test strips or paper before purchasing. On average, you can use paper rolls to test both urine and saliva, whereas single use strips are only used to test urine (but there are exceptions). Both testing methods provide an accurate picture of your pH fluctuations, however saliva testing can be a little trickier (I get to that in the upcoming section, "Testing your saliva"). Stick to whatever fluid you choose to test because saliva pH results are usually a little more acidic than urine. On average:

✔ Saliva pH ranges from 6 to 7.

✔ Urine pH ranges from 6.5 to 8.

Using test kits

Regardless of whether you use a piece of paper from a pH test roll or a pH strip, you can only use it once. You cannot reuse the test paper.

If you have strips, don't touch the colored end. If you have a roll, don't touch the end you use to dip in urine or saliva. Doing so can potentially affect your results, since you have a fine acidic layer on your skin.

Using a urine test kit

I find that urine testing is easier than saliva testing, as it provides less chance for user-error. To complete a pH urine test:

1. **Remove one test strip or rip a three-inch piece off of the roll.**

2. **Begin to urinate and release about two seconds worth of urine.**

   Your initial urine may be more acidic from sitting in your urethra, so let a couple seconds go by.

3. **Place the piece of paper or strip directly in the urine stream until it is thoroughly moistened.**

4. **Check the results immediately by comparing the color on your strip or paper to the keyed color chart on your bottle or in your packaging.**

5. **The pH number that best corresponds to your color is your urine pH right now.**

6. **Write down your results.**

   I explain how and why you want to keep a record of your results in "Monitoring Your Results" later in this chapter.

Testing your saliva

If you're squeamish about testing the pH in your urine, you can opt to test your saliva's pH. There's a catch, though — saliva testing is not as accurate in reflecting how your body dumps acids. Unlike urine testing, you also have to prepare a little before testing your saliva. You cannot test right after:

- ✔ Brushing your teeth
- ✔ Chewing gum
- ✔ Eating or drinking
- ✔ Smoking

Optimally, wait one to two hours after any of these activities , or you may end up testing the pH of whatever you ate, drank, or brushed your teeth with and get a false reading.

Know what type of water you have?

Contrary to common thought, your home tap water may not have a neutral pH. In fact, many homes have extremely alkaline water, also called *hard water,* or very acidic water, better known as *soft water.* Either extreme is bad for your plumbing, but very acidic water may also contain contaminants that can be harmful to your health after years of ingestion. Depending on your water source, these contaminants can potentially include:

- Bacteria such as E. coli

- Bromate, a chemical created during water treatment process at plants

- Haloacetic acid, a byproduct of water treatment and disinfecting

- Lead, copper, arsenic, cadmium, chromium

- Disinfectants, such as chlorine

- Radioactive particles called *radionuclides*

The health repercussions of drinking acidic water over years run the gamut from cancer to nerve damage. You can contact your water supplier and request a water quality report, which will include a list of any known contaminants (and the concentrations) in your water.

You can test the pH of your tap water with pH test strips or paper. Turn on the faucet (any one will do), hold the strip or paper under the running water and compare the color on the strip to the color on the color key. Water with a pH less than 6.5 is very acidic, whereas water with a pH greater than 8.5 is very alkaline. If you find either extreme in your home, a consultation with your water supplier is in order. You may need a water softener for extremely hard water to avoid scaling and damage to pipes.

If your tap water is not pH balanced, you may taste or see the difference. Alkaline water tastes very bitter (it's essentially mineral water) and can leave mineral scales on dishes and glass shower doors. Acidic water may have a metallic taste and cause detergents (soap, shampoo) to foam up excessively (makes you feel slimy as you exit the shower).

To test your saliva's pH:

1, **Remove one test strip or rip a three-inch piece off of the roll.**

2. **Let a little saliva gather in your mouth and spit it out, then do it again.**

    Spitting helps make sure that you test a fresh supply of saliva and not the bacteria on your teeth (yeah, yeah, we all have bacteria in our mouth).

3. **Catch a healthy portion of fresh saliva on a plastic spoon or in a small glass.**

4. **Place the piece of paper or strip directly in the saliva until it is thoroughly moistened.**

5. **Check the results immediately by comparing the color on your strip or paper to the keyed color chart on your bottle or in your packaging.**

    The pH number that best corresponds to your color is your saliva pH.

6. Write down your results for reference (I'll tell you why in this chapter).

Do *not* place the test strip or paper in your mouth — it's covered in chemical reactive agents and not at all good for you.

Checking food and beverages

At some point, you may wish to check the pH of a food or beverage. It's fun to do as long as you remember that the pH of a food going in does not equate to its potential to form acids or bases in your body. Think about sugar — it is not acidic by nature, but it is acid-forming in your body.

To check the pH of any liquid, follow the instructions in the preceding sections for checking urine or saliva pH with one exception: do not dip a test strip or paper directly into the container, especially if it's a beverage. You don't want the chemicals on the strip soaking into something you plan on drinking.

Testing solid food is a little trickier. The pH strips and paper can only detect the pH of liquids, not solids. You have the option of purchasing a pH testing meter, but only if you have hundreds of dollars to spend on this science project (they average about 250 U.S. dollars).

If you have neutral water (pH of 7) you can cheat and make your solids a liquid, but it's not the most scientifically accurate method. However, if you want to give it a whirl:

1. **Cut off a small piece of the solid food.**

2. **Place it in a blender with equal parts pH-neutral water.**

3. **Mix on high or until the solid food is liquefied.**

4. **Dip the litmus paper or strip into the liquefied food.**

5. **Compare with the color chart provided by the manufacturer and determine the pH of the food.**

Monitoring Your Results

After you know how to test your pH, you need to know a little more about what those results mean. Say you test your pH for the first time and it's 7.5 — yay, that's good right? Does that mean you're alkaline and doing a great job without even making any changes to diet or lifestyle? Maybe not, and here's why: Your pH fluctuates throughout the day as your body compensates for acid production. If you eat a cheeseburger for lunch and check your urine pH immediately afterward, you'll get a false alkaline reading because the acids from the cheeseburger haven't had a chance to run through your system yet.

You may feel the effect of the acids (heartburn, bloating) before your urine reflects an acid dump by way of a low pH. For most people, urine pH doesn't reflect that cheeseburger until later in the night (like around bedtime) or even tomorrow morning.

Selecting test times

There are right times and wrong times to test your pH. Optimally, you test your pH at the same time every day.

For the most accurate reflection of your pH, you can establish a pH baseline by testing first thing in the morning (or upon waking, if you work the night shift). Your baseline lets you see where your pH started, which can help illustrate how your diet affects your overall pH. Wow — a diet with actual, measurable health-promoting results, how great is that?

While you sleep, your kidneys filter out acids, which is why a first-thing morning urine test is most reflective of your true pH balance. Testing later in the day, like before lunch, shows a more alkaline pH — because all the acids were filtered and excreted earlier that morning. It's like leaning on the counter while you stand on the scale — sure, the numbers will look better, but it's a false representation of your true weight.

If you don't want to test your urine, remember that saliva doesn't reflect the work of your kidneys overnight. However, an early morning pH reading of your saliva is more accurate than those taken later in the day as the bacteria, food, and beverages of the day are not reflected in the morning pH result.

Yuck, that's in my mouth?

Did your mom ever chastise you for sucking on a fresh paper cut? She was right. Well over 200 types of bacteria live and thrive in the human mouth, which means you just spiced up that little paper cut with a hoard of germs. Your mouth provides a nice, warm, and wet environment for these bugs. Add in the fact that your saliva is slightly acidic, and it's like rolling out the welcome mat for bacteria.

Although you can't see them with the naked eye, these germs are ever-present and love to hibernate along the gum line in the form of plaque. *Plaque* is composed of the sticky remnants of food, saliva, and germs — getting rid of it is the reason you brush your teeth. Left unchecked, plaque causes tooth decay and gum disease — the absolute nemesis to a bright, white smile.

Testing frequency

I suggest testing your pH once daily to establish a baseline. After reading the instructions that come with your test kit, you may wonder why they tell you to test your pH three to five times daily and I tell you to only test once, maybe twice a day tops. The reason lies in a difference in perspective between the test paper manufacturers and me. From their perspective, the more you test, the more paper or strips you use — meaning you'll have to order or buy more pH test strips sooner. It's marketing at its best! Use our strips often and buy more, please. I'd prefer you save money while gauging the effects of your diet on your acid-alkaline balance.

You can choose from two methods when it comes to testing frequency:

- ✔ **Once a day:**. Test your pH once daily, every day, and watch the trends. If your pH maintains relatively stable, you may want to consider dropping test frequency to every other day to save money on strips.

- ✔ **Twice a day:** If your pH is all over the map, you can check it twice daily and take the average of your readings for a daily pH.

You can check your pH as often as you like, but the myriad results won't reflect your body's true balance.

It will take time, but over a period of weeks you should start to see a trend that becomes more alkaline in the morning (meaning your body is not working as hard to dump excess acids while you sleep). If you really want to test more frequently, you can check your pH in the morning and in the evening, right before bed. At any other time (lunch, afternoon, whenever) your body is compensating for an acidic pH — so a test only reflects an alkaline pH as your body dumps out buffers (minerals such as calcium) to neutralize the acidic pH. These false-alkaline test results may lead you in the wrong direction, thinking everything is groovy when in reality it's not.

Choosing testing mediums

Okay, I admit I'm biased on this one — I strongly encourage testing urine pH, not saliva. In my opinion, urine pH is much more reflective of your overall balance. (I tell you how in the previous section, "Using a urine test kit.") Unlike your urine, saliva pH can give false readings based on:

- ✔ Your oral health and hygiene

- ✔ The presence of yeast or bacteria

- ✔ Habits such as smoking or chewing gum

- ✔ Medical problems such as allergies or *rhinitis,* an inflammation of mucous membranes in the nose)

- ✔ If you chronically breathe through your mouth (you're what's known as a *mouth breather*), your mouth dries out, which stops saliva from washing away bacteria

- ✔ User error — if you don't get rid of all the toothpaste, food, or beverage in your mouth prior to doing a pH test, you're testing the pH of the toothpaste, food, or beverage.

One caveat: If you have chronic (or current) urinary tract infections, your urine pH may reflect the bacteria, hoards of cranberry juice you drink to get rid of the infection, or even the medicines you take for said infection.

Deciphering your results

The opinions (and there are oh so many to choose from) about the acceptable pH range of urine or saliva vary. Little to no scientific guidance states exactly where your urine pH should be at any given time. However, scientific research shows that extremes (acidic or alkaline) are not good for your body.

Consistent readings less than 6.5 are very acidic. Although you may see a few weeks of acidity while you begin the acid alkaline diet, it should not persist for months. Likewise, consistent readings above 8.0 are very alkaline — your body could be in a state of *catabolism,* which means it's breaking down lean muscle mass to combat starvation or a disease process. Either extreme should solicit a conversation with your family doctor.

On average, a normal pH ranges from 6.5 to 8.0. Your morning readings don't need to stick at 8.0 (very alkaline), but they should be more alkaline than acidic, on average. This slightly alkaline state is where your body functions at its peak, the way it was intended to work.

If your pH tests are consistently acidic (less than 7.0), you may want to consider an 80/20 diet — where 80 percent of your foods are alkaline-forming and only 20 percent are acid-forming. Once your daily pH becomes slightly alkaline (greater than 7.0) you can consider cutting back to a 60/40 diet, where 60 percent of your foods are alkaline and up to 40 percent are acid-forming. Refer to Chapter 2 if you want to review the different dietary balances to correct pH imbalances.

Interpreting variations

I know it's going to be hard, but try not to read too much into your first few pH test results. This is a time when it's good to write it down and forget it — don't harp on yourself about it. The first time I checked my morning pH I thought, "No way, *that* can't be right." During the first few weeks of a pH balanced diet, your body might appear overly alkaline or acidic — these wacky readings are the product of hitting your virtual reset button — prepare to take your body off of autopilot and resume control.

For this reason, I encourage everyone to keep a pH journal to monitor their progress and the changes that occur. You can't fix a problem until you become aware of it!

Use the information you gather to better yourself, not to get disgruntled about that glass of wine you had yesterday.

Keeping a Journal

I am a visual learner — the best way to monitor my pH results and attribute them to diet, exercise, and changes in my lifestyle is by looking at a graph. (I know, nerd alert, right?) It actually isn't that difficult to chart your pH, and a journal can help you find your personal hot spots — things that you could change now to affect your health later.

Logging entries

You'll need a few cheap supplies (or a computer) to get started. Personally, I track my pH on a Microsoft Excel spreadsheet — but unless you're computer savvy, that will add more frustration than is necessary. If you're going to journal by hand (the easiest way) you need:

- A notebook and pencil
- Graph paper

Consider logging entries that include your:

- pH result and the date and time of the result
- Diet (everything you eat or drink)
- Symptoms throughout the day (be specific!)
- Activity levels and time

Figure 4-1 shows a few days of a food journal.

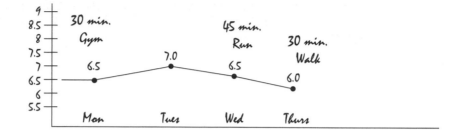

Monday

a.m. pH 6.5
Breakfast: Tofu scramble, 8oz. almond milk, sm. banana
Lunch: Shrimp salad, steamed broccoli
Snacks: Lemon water, handful almonds
Dinner: 3oz. salmon, spinach salad, sprouted grain roll

Tuesday

a.m. pH 7.0
Breakfast: Whey smoothie with granola
Lunch: Egg white asparagus omelet
Snacks: Popcorn, kale chips
Dinner: 3oz. chicken & spelt pasta

Wednesday

a.m. pH 6.5
Breakfast: 1 egg white, 8oz. almond milk, granola
Lunch: Gazpacho, sprouted tortilla, lemon water
Snacks: Grilled fruit, kale chips & salsa
Dinner: Tofu Stir fry

Thursday

Figure 4-1:
Food journal
entries and
plotted pH
readings.

a.m. pH 6.0
Breakfast: Tofu scramble
Lunch: Veggie pizza
Snacks: Sm. apple, handful almonds, soy smoothie
Dinner: Stuffed green peppers

pH

Unless you want double the work, record your pH onto the graph paper the moment you take it. Mark dates along the horizontal line (if you're testing once daily) and pH values on the vertical axis. Figure 4-2 shows what my first pH graph looked like.

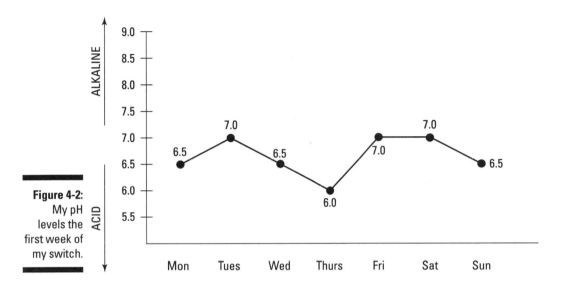

Figure 4-2:
My pH
levels the
first week of
my switch.

Symptoms

Be specific and pay attention to your body. The more in-tune you become, the less likely you are to miss a sign or symptom of acidity. Anywhere on the graph (or on a separate, dated sheet of paper in your journal) jot down specific symptoms you incur each day.

Try not to generalize ("felt yucky") as that isn't a specific symptom. Instead, consider writing, "headache for one hour" or "heartburn at 6 pm." These are distinct symptoms that you may be able to correlate to an acidic dietary impact over time.

Diet

This one may seem obvious, but it's important to log. You can jot down your daily intake on a separate sheet of journal paper or right on the graph (personally, I started by writing everything I ate and drank under the date right on the graph paper). Over time, you can see the acidic pH dips following an indulgence.

After months of balancing your pH diet, your body gets spoiled and may react harshly to the ingestion of acid-forming foods (big pH drop the following day).

Activity

Did you work out today? How hard and for how long? Write down your activity levels and watch the trends over time. You may see how vigorous exercise sessions (over one hour) drastically impact your pH the next day. This isn't an excuse to stop exercising, but to learn how to compensate for a sweaty gym session. Chapter 6 talks more about exercise, lifestyle, and pH impact.

General snapshot

How are you feeling in general today? How would you describe your mood? Energy level? Libido? Journaling about your general health and happiness provides an overall snapshot of the benefits you reap on a pH balanced diet.

Don't forget to record stray comments from loved ones, coworkers, or friends. Things like, "You look great, what are you doing different?" were a real self-confidence booster and motivator for me when I got started.

Making the connection

After you plot a few weeks of pH, symptoms, diet, and activity, you may start to see a connection among acidic dips, diet, and trends. Sometimes, this connection is quite obvious. If it isn't, pull out your highlighter, I'll show you how to connect the dots if they don't stand out.

Use a highlighter to demarcate every acidic pH on the graph. Depending on your body, you may process acids within a few hours or a few days — everyone's different in this aspect. For each highlighted pH, look to the diet and exercise prior and highlight any acid-forming suspects. If on Wednesday your pH was 6.5 in the morning, look back to Tuesday and highlight any activity, foods, or beverages that may the culprit.

Every acidic pH dip has a cause — you just have to find it. If you have exhausted all foods, beverages, and activities from the day before, consider other factors — elevated levels of stress and a lack of sleep can affect your pH. Consider adding more details to your journal in the future including:

- Hours of sleep the night prior
- Quality of sleep
- Any illness such as an impending cold or flu
- Stressors in your life (work, social obligations, and so on)

Keeping it real

Your journal is only as good as you make it. If you forget to log entries for a few days, then go back and arbitrarily throw in some values, it's a lost cause. My advice: Start fresh and take it as a lesson learned. The more accurate, detailed, and timely your journal is, the more useful it is in defining your pH balance and acid excretion problems.

Seeing the Good Stuff

Ah, my least favorite question (because the answer is so ambiguous): When will I start to see results from my pH balancing efforts? Seeing the good stuff happen occurs at different intervals for everyone depending on:

- Your level of dedication to the diet and lifestyle
- Your personal health history and any current medical problems
- Your weight and lean muscle mass
- Addictions (smoking, drinking, recreational drug use)

You should begin to witness a mix of immediate and chronic changes towards wellness. Immediate changes occur as you decrease the workload on your body, whereas chronic, or long-term changes emerge as your body repairs years of damage to cells.

Detecting immediate changes

The most common (and gratifying) changes you experience soon after decreasing your intake of acid-forming foods and adapting your lifestyle may not be obvious. You may start to wake up feeling less groggy or simply feel cheerful — and that can be just enough to keep you motivated!

The immediate benefits of the acid alkaline diet stem from a decreased workload in your body — it no longer has to work full-time to flush out all the acids. It's like giving your body a vacation! (How nice is *that*?) You may start to see:

- Increased energy and stamina
- Increased focus and memory retention
- Less digestive symptoms (heartburn, bloating)
- Regular bowel movements

When I say *immediate*, I'm not referring to time but to the type of health benefits you witness. You may not have immediate relief of constipation, but increasing regularity may be one of the first or foremost signs that your body agrees with the diet.

Watching for chronic improvement

Over time (possibly many months), a pH balanced diet, exercise, and lifestyle allows your body to store reserves of energy and fight acidity at the cellular level. This is when the great stuff starts to happen — the reduced risk of chronic diseases such as type 2 diabetes and increased immunity leading to fewer head colds and viruses. Other systems impacted over time may include:

- ✔ Weight loss and stabilization (no more yo-yoing for you!)
- ✔ Decreased generalized aches and pains
- ✔ Stabilized bone density (your body is no longer stealing calcium)
- ✔ Decreased stone formation (kidney stones, gallstones)
- ✔ Improved digestion
- ✔ Reduced risk of coronary disease, certain cancers, and stroke

After you stick with an acid alkaline diet for a few months, take a moment and consider — have you finally found your own personal fountain of youth? It may have been hiding, buried by acids, inside you all along.

Part II

Homeostasis: Keeping Your Body Happy

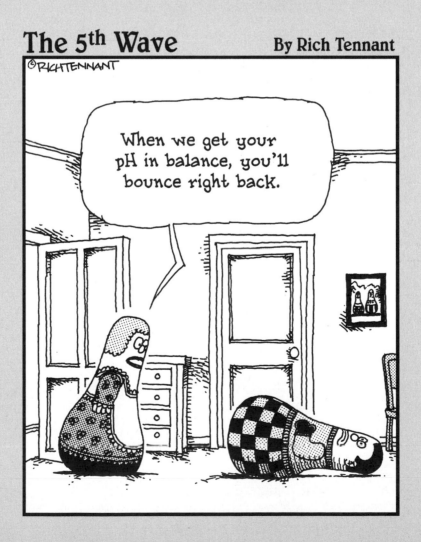

In this part...

So you've heard that diet and nutrition can impact your body's pH, but how does that work? I'm of the mind that you should understand how something works before you attempt to repair it. Every cell in your body has its own pH balance. The acid alkaline diet can't change your blood pH — only your body can do that. A pH balanced diet can reduce the work of your pH regulating systems, which helps your body function at its peak and return to its preferred alkaline state.

The chapters in this part illustrate exactly what a pH is and how your body regulates it. Everything you do — and don't do — affects your pH balance. I explain how things like diet, exercise, and even your mood can negatively impact your pH level. And I show you how to fix it.

Chapter 5

What the Heck is a pH and What Can You Do about It?

In This Chapter:

▶ Understanding pH

▶ Discovering what affects your pH

▶ Looking at ways to balance your pH

▶ Finding out how acidic you are

Your pH balance is what makes you a living, breathing, carbon-based life form. Your *pH* (technically the potential of hydrogen) is a measurement of acidity and alkalinity (base) on a 0 to 14 scale. The *pH balance* is how your body keeps the acids and bases in check. Without an intrinsic pH balance, you'd be dead.

Just as you don't have to think about breathing every few seconds, you don't have to work to control your pH. That's not to say that your body always knows what is best for you. I said you didn't *have to* control your pH, not that you wouldn't *want to*. I even wrote this book to tell you how.

This chapter explains the foundations of pH balance, and illustrates how acid and alkaline substances influence your internal environment.

Because they're one in the same, you'll see me use the terms *pH balance* and *acid base balance* interchangeably.

Explaining the pH

Your body is composed of trillions of microscopic cells. Each cell has a membrane and a pH balance. Together, your cells create your internal pH environment, which is the overall measurement of acids and bases throughout your body. This internal pH environment influences every single function in your body, from breathing to digestion.

The abbreviation *pH* stands for "potential of hydrogen" — your entire pH balance hinges on the microscopic hydrogen ion. Too much hydrogen and you become acidic, whereas a deficit makes you alkalotic.

Your body wants a slightly alkaline environment so that it can function at peak performance.

Watch for these early symptoms that you may be heading into acid-land:

- ✔ Feeling tired, groggy, irritable
- ✔ Weight gain, even after dieting
- ✔ Stomach upset and frequent digestive problems
- ✔ Hair loss
- ✔ Frequent illness

Uh-oh — did I just describe you? It's okay, I probably just described half of the people I know. But trying to solve these issues through the self-help section of the bookstore or the over-the-counter supplement section at the drugstore isn't the way to go. The answers are not rooted in psychological issues or found in a pill bottle. They are found in the basic principle of pH, or acid base, balance.

Reading the pH scale

Think of the pH scale in linear terms. Acid is at one end of the spectrum measuring 0 and alkaline on the opposite measuring 14. Your pH is almost dead center, but as Figure 5-1 shows, everybody is naturally a little alkaline.

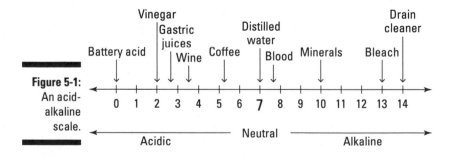

Figure 5-1:
An acid-alkaline scale.

Your pH level varies slightly depending on which bodily fluid you test, with your blood being the most sensitive to pH fluctuations. The average pH levels for bodily fluids are

- Tears = 7.20
- Blood = 7.41
- Urine = 6.5 - 8.0
- Sweat = < 6.0

Your blood prefers a static pH measurement at 7.41 (alkaline). Any deviations in your blood pH initiate a body-wide chain reaction to get back to the baseline. Excess acids are dumped out of your bloodstream and into your tissues for disposal. (On average, tissue pH ranges from 7.35 to 7.45 in a healthy person.) Extra acids leave your tissues either through your urine or your sweat.

The kidneys filter out the excess acids and BOOM — the pH measurement of your urine becomes more acidic, reflecting the fact that acids are leaving your body. Sometimes acids are excreted through your sweat as well.

Your sweat is always acidic — averaging less than 6.0 on the pH scale. This is due in part to the protective covering called the *acid mantle* — a layer of acid and wax (called *sebum*) that sits on top of your skin and repels hostile invaders such as germs. When your sweat mingles with the acid mantle, it decreases the pH of the sweat a bit.

When you try to change your pH through diet, you're talking about altering your pH as whole, not just your blood pH or tissue pH.

Similar to your blood pressure and your heart rate, your pH is a fluid measurement. I don't mean fluid as in water, I mean fluid as in ever-changing, not constant. Your pH measurements vary throughout the day. The urine pH of a healthy individual may be slightly acidic in the morning (between 6.5 and 7). After a day's worth of healthy alkaline foods, exercise, and acid buffering, your urine pH may tend to be more alkaline at bedtime (7.5-8). Ideally, you're looking for an average on the alkalotic side as opposed to always scoring acidic on the pH scale when testing your urine. (I tell you how to do that in Chapter 4.)

You may notice fluctuations throughout the day if you test the pH of your urine or saliva at different times. This is normal. Your pH fluctuates from minute to minute, similar to your heart or respiratory rate. The acid base balance is fluid — constantly changing. Thank goodness! If it weren't, there would be no way you could fix it.

Try not to (you will) over-compensate. If you are tracking your pH measurements, realize that the first few weeks of your new diet and lifestyle are a transitional phase, so let your body get used to the new environment and don't rely too heavily on the pH readings.

Reviewing just a little chemistry — acids and bases

Yeah, yeah, I hated chemistry as a kid, too. But just a couple basic chemistry concepts can help you on your journey to understanding your pH balance:

- An **acid** is any substance that measure less than 7 on the linear pH scale, to a maximum acidity of pH 0. Everything you do that uses energy — from breathing to moving to digesting — triggers acid production in your body.

  You have naturally occurring acids and alkaline substances in your body. Carbon dioxide (CO_2), the stuff you breathe out all day, is an acid.

- A **base** is an alkaline substance, the polar opposite of an acid, that measures greater than 7 to a maximum pH of 14. Also naturally produced in your body, bases substances are better known as *alkaline buffers,* meaning they buffer, or neutralize, acidity.

  Bicarbonate (HCO_3), which lives in your tissues, is your body's primary alkaline source. Bicarbonate is an alkaline substance controlled by the kidneys (absorbed or released as needed). Its main function is maintaining the acid base balance.

The back and forth between acids and alkaline buffers is how your body achieves its pH balance. (I talk about the role of buffers later in this section.)

Your naturally occurring acids, which balance out your bases, include:

- **Hydrochloric acid:** Your stomach is brimming over with hydrochloric acid — it's what digests your food. Hydrochloric acid has a pH around 2.0.

  Ever get heartburn? It's more accurately called *acid reflux* and is a symptom of your stomach acid burbling up your esophagus. You get acid reflux when you eat too many acidic foods, such as citrus, or as a symptom of a *stomach ulcer* (an open sore in the lining of the stomach).

- **Lactic acid:** Lactic acid is produced when you use energy to move. When you wiggle your fingers, your cells kick on to make energy. The byproduct of that energy is lactic acid. Unfortunately, it's a bit like the exhaust from your car as you speed down the highway — necessary but yucky in that too much lactic acids building up in your tissues can cause pain. Lactic acid has a pH around 3.0.

✔ **Carbonic acid:** Sometime within the last five seconds you have exhaled a breath. That is your body getting rid of carbonic acid, which is dissolved in the carbon dioxide you exhale. This acid is the byproduct of respiration (also known as breathing). Oxygen floods into your lungs and is transported to every cell in your body via your blood. The waste — carbon dioxide and acids — is transported back to your lungs to be released. Carbonic acid has a pH around 5.0.

The bases, which neutralize the acids in your body, include:

✔ **Calcium:** Calcium is stored throughout your body — in your bones, teeth, blood — even at the cellular level. This mineral is a potent fountain of alkalinity within your body. It is known as a *pH buffer,* which means that it is leeched from your tissues and released into your bloodstream when your pH becomes too acidic. This leeching process is good for your blood, but bad for your bones — another reason to keep your pH level in check. Calcium has a pH around 9.0 to 10.0.

✔ **Bicarbonate:** You probably know this as baking soda, but bicarbonate is present throughout your body and mainly stored in the kidneys. Bicarbonate is another big buffer used by your body to control pH. When you eat acid-forming foods, your body releases stores of bicarbonate to regulate your pH. This process is not as fast as your respiratory control, and it can take days to neutralize *acidic ash,* which is the acidic residue left in your digestive system. Bicarbonate has a pH around 10.0.

✔ **Potassium and magnesium:** Potassium and magnesium are minerals that leave an *alkaline ash,* or an *alkaline residue,* within your body. They are also integral to your personal electrical system, having a symbiotic relationship with calcium that helps you control your muscles. Since your heart is a muscle, these nutrients are vital to controlling your heart rate. They average a pH around 9.0 to 10.0.

Table 5-1 puts the acids and bases and their functions in an easy-to-read format:

Table 5-1		Acids and Bases in Your Body	
Acid	*Function*	*Base*	*Function*
Hydrochloric acid	Digestion	Calcium	Bones and fluid balance
Lactic acid	Energy byproduct	Bicarbonate	Neutralize acids
Carbonic acid	Respiration	Potassium and magnesium	Fluid balance

Making the energy-acid connection

Your body always needs energy. Even while you sit reading this, your body is creating and burning energy to:

- ✔ Digest food
- ✔ Filter blood
- ✔ Inflate your lungs
- ✔ Move waste through your small intestine and colon
- ✔ Produce urine
- ✔ Pump your heart
- ✔ Regulate your temperature

Shall I go on? I'm exhausted just reading the list. While your body is doing all of these splendid, life-sustaining things, it's creating a byproduct of acid.

As your body produces energy, it also produces acid — it's as simple as that. The more active you are, the more energy you need. Although you use energy as you exercise, the movement stimulates a chemical reaction, telling your brain to make more energy for sustained movement.

Influencing Your pH

You influence your pH balance through dietary and lifestyle choices. Your little choices (it's always the small things that count) directly impact your pH fluctuations.

Many factors affect your pH balance. Just as you can't fly a plane without learning about the controls, you can't pilot your body's pH without learning about all the things that impact your balancing act.

What you eat clearly plays a large role in helping you regulate your acid intake, but aside from diet, your lifestyle choices —couch potato versus wonder woman, smoker versus non-smoker, and whether you drink more water than alcohol — have a huge impact on your health.

You cannot control the regulation mechanisms in play *after* you ingest acid-forming foods, which is why adhering to an acid-alkaline diet is so important.

The following sections explain the good and bad ways to deal with the major factors affecting pH. You can find out more about reducing the impacts of exercise and non-dietary pH choices in Chapter 6.

What you eat

Skeptics will tell you that you cannot influence your pH through diet because all alkaline substances are destroyed in the gastric (hydrochloric) acid of your stomach during digestion. Hogwash! After you eat an acid-forming food, your pH level falls down the scale and becomes acidic.

I'm not going to drive this point home with any cheesy cliché such as, *you are what you eat* (oops, I just said it, didn't I?), but I will say that your dietary choices make the biggest impact on your pH balance. Certain foods, including animal proteins, refined and wheat grains, and sugars leave an acidic ash in your digestive tract. This drops your pH and turns your tissues acidic (a little something I refer to as *entering acid land*). Your cells cannot thrive in an acidic environment — too much acid leads to cellular death and illness. You can go to Chapter 2 if you want a more specific food list.

Conversely, choosing foods that leave an alkaline ash helps keep your pH out of the acid range. Your body is at its happiest when your pH is slightly alkaline. Almost every plant food (in its natural state) *is* alkaline. The big exception here is starchy veggies and grains — wheat, refined flour, corn, and white potatoes. These grains and vegetables have a high natural sugar content, which leaves an acidic ash in your body.

What you drink

The fluids you drink (or don't drink) have a huge impact on your pH. If you like a lot of carbonation and drink sodas all day long, you're drinking carbonic acid, which acidifies your body. It takes gallons of fresh water to flush out the carbonic acid of just one soda.

Water intake is directly linked to your pH balance. It's so vital, in fact, that I dedicate an entire section to water in Chapter 6. If you don't drink enough (at least eight, 8-ounce glasses each day), the acids can't move out of your tissues. Water is a transporter, flushing out these acids and carrying them to your skin and urine, where your get rid of them.

A word on coffee, tea, and alcohol: These beverages dehydrate you. Ever run to the bathroom after a cup of coffee or a bottle of beer? These fluids are known as *diuretics* (or what grandma calls her water pill), which steal water from your tissues and send you to the bathroom every five minutes. Although I give you some tips on how to continue enjoying coffee and tea in Chapter 6, try to avoid alcohol altogether because it is very acidifying.

What you do

Although it would be wonderful if I could say that following an acid alkaline diet means you don't have to exercise, I can't.

Aside from what you eat, the way you approach physical fitness (and your current fitness level) has a huge impact on your pH balance. Consider what exercise does for your body:

- ✔ Improves cardiovascular function and circulation
- ✔ Assists with weight control
- ✔ Increases your energy production
- ✔ Releases chemicals that make you happy

Now, consider how these functions impact your pH. It takes longer for the couch potato to flush out acids than it does in an active person. If you are overweight, acids have more places to hide in your body (they have an affinity for fat cells). If you exercise routinely, your body does not have to work as hard making more energy — it becomes highly adept at the process. The happy chemicals — they don't impact your pH so much, but they can impact your state of mind.

If you're just starting an exercise program, jumping in headfirst to a strenuous daily workout is a huge pH no-no. You need to exercise at least 20 to 30 minutes per day, but there is a right way to get started to help your body decrease its acidic buildup and learn how to use oxygen (using oxygen is what burns fat, by the way) to power your body. Chapter 6 has all the details on how to exercise the right way.

If you're not fit and push your body during exercise, three things happen simultaneously that contribute to an acid build-up:

- ✔ You start to breath shallowly, causing a build-up of carbon dioxide (acid) in your lungs.
- ✔ The cellular components that create energy (mitochondria) release an acid byproduct as they try to fuel your muscles.
- ✔ Your body switches into an *anaerobic metabolism* and starts to burn your cells' energy sources instead of oxygen. This process creates a byproduct of more lactic acid and cellular waste.

  Have your muscles ever burned badly after a workout? It was caused by a buildup of lactic acid from your anaerobic metabolism.

Burning oxygen during a workout is desirable — that's good aerobic exercise — but stealing your cell's food supply by pushing your body to an anaerobic state is not.

What you don't do

I'm not going to tell you that quitting smoking is easy, because it isn't. But it *is* vital to your pH balance — and your health in general. Talk to your doctor if you need help to quit. Tobacco use acidifies you by:

- ✔ Cellular damage from the cigarette chemicals create acid.
- ✔ The nicotine decreases your circulation, which means acids take longer to get out of your system.
- ✔ Tobacco alters the pH in your mouth, which can lead to gum disease, cavities, and bad breath (germs thrive in the acid).

Can you see the vicious cycle starting here? Whether you chew tobacco or smoke it, it will continue to unbalance your pH.

Although I touch on the sugar in relation to vegetables and starches in the previous "What you eat" section, many different kinds of sugar can acidify your body. As you'll see in the recipes I provide in Part 4, sugars are a pH no-no and should be avoided including:

- ✔ Aspartame
- ✔ Honcy
- ✔ Granulated, brown, and powdered sugars
- ✔ Any artificial sweetener (excluding Stevia, which has minimal pH impact)

Seeking Balance

When your pH balance becomes too acidic, you create an unstable environment that is susceptible to waste build up and cellular death. Imagine if you never took the trash out of your home again. It would eventually become uninhabitable, right? The same thing occurs in your body. An acidic environment kills your cells, which in turn die and build up as waste throughout your body. This waste piles up and can start to impact your overall health, starting with feeling generally off (tired, cranky) leading to illness (frequent colds). See Chapter 3 to learn more about the impacts of acidity in your body.

If left unbalanced, an acidic environment has a corrosive effect in your body. Imagine putting watered-down gasoline in a sports car. The car will run, but over time, the parts get corroded and start causing big bills at the auto mechanic. Your body is not that different from the sports car. When you're too far over on one side of the acid-alkaline scale, your body works hard behind the scenes to re-establish that vital pH balance — using up precious resources and energy in the process. Why make your body work so hard if you don't have to?

If you continue to dump acids into your system, your pH balance will suffer and stay acidic. Your body may still be dealing with the pH disturbance from yesterday's yummy yeasty rolls — it hasn't even had a chance to deal with the donuts you had for breakfast today!

If you are currently partaking in SAD, better known as the Standard American Diet, rife with fat, sugar, and carbs, there is very little chance of overdoing it on the alkaline side of the scale.

Figure 5-2 illustrates how many times Joseph impacted his pH in one day. Coffee with sugar and creamer? Acid with acid and acid. Bagel? More acid in the form of refined grains and sugary carbs. He's piling on the acids and it's not even noon!

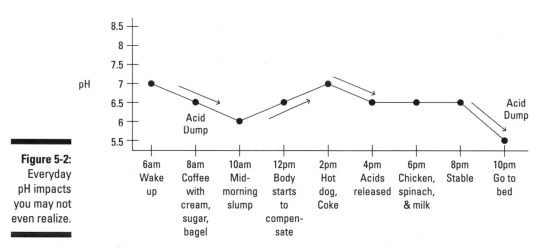

Figure 5-2:
Everyday pH impacts you may not even realize.

Looking at your regulation mechanisms

Your body has a system of checks and balances in place — it is constantly working to keep your pH balanced. No matter what else is going on with your body, if you're walking and talking, two systems are busy maintaining your blood pH for you:

- ✔ Your lungs retain or exhale carbonic acid.
- ✔ Your kidneys retain or release bicarbonate.

The kidneys and lungs function in harmony — like a system of check and balances — to physiologically alter your pH levels and to correct an imbalanced pH.

The technical term for this regulation of pH is *compensation.* You have an acid build-up because you're exercising? You may start breathing a little faster to blow off some carbonic acid in your carbon dioxide . You're a little too alkaline because you just witnessed a car accident and started to hyperventilate (exhaling too much acid, too fast)? Your kidneys reabsorb some bicarbonate (alkaline), and your brain slows your breathing rate.

Figure 5-3 shows the symbiotic relationship of your brain, lungs, and kidneys with pH.

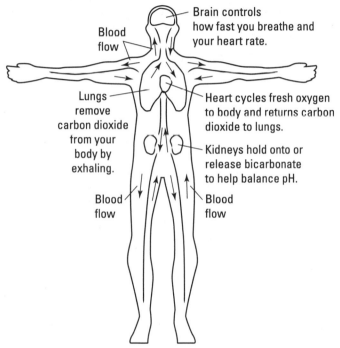

Brain controls how fast you breathe and your heart rate.

Blood flow

Lungs remove carbon dioxide from your body by exhaling.

Heart cycles fresh oxygen to body and returns carbon dioxide to lungs.

Kidneys hold onto or release bicarbonate to help balance pH.

Blood flow

Blood flow

Figure 5-3:
How the carbon dioxide exchange works.

You are not in control of your blood pH. Only your brain regulates that.

To fully understand your pH regulation, you must first understand how your nervous system controls your pH. Your nervous system is composed of two parts:

- The **central nervous system** includes your brain, spinal cord, and the little chemical messengers that circulate your body (neurons).

- The **peripheral nervous system** is composed of pretty much everything else — cranial nerves, spinal nerves, even the nerve endings in your fingers.

    The peripheral nervous system controls homeostasis and therefore, pH.

I've got the vapors

Ever sit and wonder why you breathe? What caused all those big screen heroines to get "the vapors"? Your carbonic acid plays a key role in keeping your breathing regular. Your central nervous system sends a signal to your brain that your acid levels are increasing (retaining too much carbonic acid). In turn, your brain shoots a message to the diaphragm and stimulates a breath. Carbonic acid dissolves within the lungs (in carbon dioxide) and is exhaled out with a breath, resetting the pH balance. Don't believe me? Go sprint up a flight of stairs. Did you start breathing heavily? Your body was trying to blow off the excess acids to maintain your pH. When women get "the vapors", they were either hyperventilating or holding their breath — getting their pH and carbonic acids out of whack. Ultimately, your body will fix it by making you pass out!

Your central and peripheral nervous systems work behind the scenes regulating your:

- **Blood pressure:** Peripheral nervous system receptors in your blood vessels tell your brain how "stretched" your blood vessels are. More stretch equals lower blood pressure, whereas tight, constricted vessels cause higher blood pressure.

- **Heart rate:** Your nervous system tells your brain when there is too little or too much blood circulating through your heart, which results in an increased or decreased heart rate.

- **Metabolism:** Metabolism is the collective term for every single chemical reaction occurring in your body at once, including the production of energy, digestion, and even the breakdown of injured or dead cells. Your endocrine system (hormones) and nerves work together to regulate your metabolic rate (how fast or slow your metabolism works) and decide how efficiently your body needs to be run.

- **pH balance:** Your pH balance is influenced by positive and negative feedback from peripheral nerves throughout your body. Your peripheral nerves send messages (*feedback*) to your central nervous system — "Hey, the blood in these fingertips is too acidic" and your brain makes the corresponding adjustment, "Hey heart, beat a little faster and flush out that acid!" Your pH balance controls everything from breathing to digestion — including the health and function of every cell in your body.

- **Temperature:** Billions of nerve endings in your skin tell your brain if you are too cold or warm, trying to constantly keep your thermostat around 98.6 degrees Fahrenheit. Your peripheral nerve endings work with your central nervous system (brain) to regulate your temperature.

Take a deep breath. You just overrode your peripheral nervous system! These processes are *involuntary,* which means you do not have to control them, but you can influence them. Table 5-2 shows the involuntary processes and how you can manipulate them consciously.

So, why do you need to know about all these voluntary and involuntary functions? They help you to better understand your body, and how *everything* you do impacts your pH levels. Eat a donut? Become acidic. Get mad and start yelling? Become acidic. Stop going to the gym and sit on the couch? Become acidic. If you understand how these functions impact your pH, you can be more cognizant of them throughout each day.

Table 5-2	Controlling Involuntary Functions
Involuntary Function	*Controllable Influences*
pH balance	Eating acid-forming foods, taking medications for heartburn, doing prolonged exercise, smoking, drinking alcohol, breathing fast or slow
Heart rate	Excitement, anger, fear, holding your breath, exercise, dehydration
Blood pressure	Anger, fear, excitement, dehydration, over-hydration, exercise
Temperature	Exercise, donning or removing clothes, fanning yourself, taking a warm bath or a cold shower
Metabolism	Exercise, nutrition

Giving your body feedback

You can help regulate your pH by understanding what makes it tick. Homeostasis is your thermostat for pH control.

Your pH balance is the cornerstone of *homeostasis,* the ongoing process that balances your *internal environment* (everything under your skin: think cells, liquids, tissues) using positive and negative feedback mechanisms and your central nervous system. Put simply: If you're cold, you shiver; if you're hot, you sweat. This is homeostasis in action — your body on autopilot. Most of the time, this process keeps things on an even keel. However, autopilot isn't always the best option when it comes to your pH or your diet.

Who thought up the word *homeostasis*?

The word homeostasis actually comes from the Greek. The prefix *homeo* means "same, unchanging, static." The suffix *–stasis* translates to "standing," so *homeostasis* is loosely translated to "standing unchanged."

Sir Walter Cannon coined the term *homeostasis* in 1933. He was trying to find a superior word to describe the body's internal balance, and he found the word *equilibria* lacking.

Claude Bernard explored the concept of *milieu interier* — regulating the internal environment, or what we now know as homeostasis — in the 1800s through his teaching about the concepts of the interior and exterior human environment and impacts. (He was also the first to establish the functions of sugar metabolism in the liver — but that's a whole other book!)

Homeostasis is not something you can control — it is an innate function constantly working behind the scenes. What you *can* control is how much acid you dump into your system — and ease the behind the scenes workload on your body.

In terms of biological feedback, positive does not mean "good" and negative does not equal "bad." Positive feedback amplifies a situation in your body whereas negative feedback returns things to baseline. Shivering when you are chilly is a result of your nervous system recognizing that you are cold. The negative feedback is the shivering, which should generate heat and bring your core temperature back to normal. Milk production when a mother is breastfeeding is an example of positive feedback. The baby suckles, more milk is created, more milk is released.

You use your body's defenses for your own good when you make the switch to an acid alkaline diet by using negative feedback. When you stop feeding your tissues acids, your body can fine-tune your pH balance from there, instead of constantly working to fix a chronic imbalance. Your body likes an alkaline environment. If you are too acidic, cells start to die.

Natural homeostasis gets you only so far — you will stay alive, but will you be healthful? Energized? Disease-free? You can be if you maintain a healthy pH balance.

Discovering How Acidic Your Lifestyle Is

Scientific advances continue to echo one principle: You are what you eat. The choices you make impact your health, plain and simple. To further complicate matters, the modern lifestyle is fraught with acidity. You may be bombarded daily with high-stress environments, less time for leisure, and a society where red meat and sugary carbs are dietary staples.

You can't fix anything until you know it is broken. Imagine how many people are probably walking around acidic right now. Consider all of the complaints you've had over the last month or so. Have you felt tired? Are weight-loss strategies failing? Do you get ill frequently? There is a chance that these innocuous sounding complaints are related to one fixable component — your pH level imbalance.

Every question in the following quiz is designed to test your *affinity* for acid, or how naturally attracted you are to a lifestyle that promotes acidity.

If you have already tested your pH level, the acidic result is not worth focusing on right now. Instead, focus on your pH lifestyle *baseline*, or the starting point illustrating the factors that led up to the acidic result.

Read each question carefully, selecting the choice that best fits your lifestyle and daily choices (not the choices you wish you made). Compare your answers to the scoring key at the end of this section to see your acid affinity.

   1. How many times a week do you eat red or processed meat?

       A. Daily

       B. Two or more times

       C. Once

       D. Never, I don't eat red or processed meat

   2. How many fresh fruits and vegetables do you eat daily?

       A. I don't eat plant food

       B. Rarely

       C. Probably two to three a day

       D. I eat more than five servings daily

3. How often do you exercise?

    A. I don't exercise

    B. Once a week

    C. Two or three times weekly

    D. Between five and seven days a week

4. Do you smoke cigarettes or use tobacco?

    A. Yes, daily

    B. Socially, a few times a week

    C. I recently quit

    D. I do not smoke or use tobacco

5. How much water do you drink a day?

    A. I do not drink water

    B. Maybe one or two glasses

    C. Between four and five glasses

    D. I drink at least eight, eight ounce glasses of water

6. How often do you eat sweets?

    A. Every time I get a chance

    B. Daily

    C. Maybe once a week

    D. Infrequently, only for special occasions

7. How frequently do you eat refined grains? (white bread, white or brown rice, cake)

    A. With every meal

    B. Daily

    C. Between two and four times a week

    D. Rarely

8. How often do you consume alcohol?

    A. A few drinks daily

    B. Two or three times a week

    C. Socially only

    D. Rarely, or I abstain from alcohol altogether

Give yourself three points for each question you answered with an "A," two points for each "B," one point for each "C," and zero points for each "D." Add up your total score and find your base in the following list:

- ✔ **0 to 5:** Congratulations! You're living a low-acid lifestyle. Keep up the great work.

- ✔ **6 to 11:** Good job, you're well on your way to a low-acid lifestyle. Examine the areas where you scored higher to start implementing positive changes in your diet or lifestyle.

- ✔ **12 to 18:** Your lifestyle or diet is contributing to an acidic environment. Look at the questions you answered with an "A" or "B"; these are the areas you can focus on immediately to improve.

- ✔ **19 to 24:** Your lifestyle and diet indicate that you're living an extremely acidic lifestyle. Consider retaking the test after a month on the acid alkaline diet to see your scores improve.

Don't fret if your quiz illustrated a very acidic lifestyle — it can only get better from here! Now that you're starting to recognize the impact of acids in your life, you can prepare yourself to make a change.

Chapter 6

Finding Some Balance in Your pH and Your Life

I'd love to say that a pH balanced diet alone can rock your world and create a healthier version of you — but that'd be a bold-faced lie. Myriad forces affect your pH balance alongside what you eat. This chapter builds upon your pH expertise by explaining the additional work needed for your body to balance itself under stress.

As a living, breathing organism, everything you do (or don't do) impacts your body. Your health hinges upon the choices you make day after day. Some choices, like when you decide to quit smoking, have an immediate impact. Other choices — cheesecake or a brisk walk — may not seem so gratifying at first, but they are equally important.

Have you heard of the Taoist concept of yin and yang? Everything in the universe has a delicate, natural balance. The two principles, yin and yang, must co-exist to exist at all. To day there is night, to good there is evil, and to acid there is alkaline — an alkaline environment is required to sustain life but all of life's sustaining functions create acid.

This chapter is for everyone like me, who will try to rationalize why X or Y is still okay on the acid alkaline diet. Been there, done that — like when I started a certain low-carbohydrate, high-protein diet and rationalized that a taco was probably acceptable because it contained beef and cheese.

Abandoning a Sedentary Lifestyle

It's not going to be easy to break out of a sedentary lifestyle, or one where you have little to no physical activity. Having said that, exercising is one of the healthiest things you can do for your body. Exercise has many benefits including:

- Weight loss or stabilization
- Increased lean muscle mass
- Improving heart and lung function
- Increased balance, coordination, and stamina
- Increased self esteem and confidence
- Decreased stress (and stress response)
- Promoting healthy sleep patterns
- Elevating mood naturally
- Removing toxins
- Circulating nutrients to the body

Wow, that's quite a list, right? Now I'm going to drop the other shoe — if done improperly, exercise can actually increase your acidity and stress out your body. In my opinion, this is the number one reason all of those New Years resolutions are destined to fail. When you push your body too hard, you actually start to feel worse. The result? You stop working out and drop your New Years resolution, returning to the safe and comfortable norm of doing nothing.

Appreciating the impact of exercise

The minute you start any kind of physical activity, several things occur simultaneously:

- Your heart rate speeds up to shuttle extra oxygen and nutrients to your muscles.
- Your muscles turn on and begin burning up the oxygen to create energy for contractions.
- Your lungs cue in on the excess acids building up, your respiratory rate picks up, and you start to breath faster.

All of these escalating functions drive up your internal temperature and you start to sweat (your body's natural way of cooling you back down to a safe temperature).

There are two types of exercise: aerobic and anaerobic. Aerobic exercise improves cardiovascular function and overall health by steadily using oxygen to help feed muscles. Anaerobic exercise is a throwback from your caveman ancestors — it allows for quick, extreme bursts of energy by creating (and burning) a sugar called *pyruvate*.

Your body turns pyruvate into lactate, which fuels the muscles (like high octane) for the short term. The byproduct of this energy burst is lactic acid. Your body cannot sustain anaerobic exercise very long — around one to three minutes tops. This is the energy production system that allows adults to lift cars during an emergency or a weight lifter to dead lift 500 pounds during a competition.

There is a happy ending here. The more you exercise, the more your body adapts to the increased demands you place on it. Over time, your heart and lungs become more efficient and stronger, which means you can exercise longer and harder with less anaerobic involvement.

Less anaerobic involvement equals less acid production and healthier exercise. You train your body to stop the anaerobic metabolism and use the aerobic metabolism by gradually building up your exercise.

Save your money

Unless you really, really want to, you don't have to spend your money on fancy leotards or gym memberships. You don't even need to buy exercise equipment. If you get creative, you can exercise using whatever you find in your home. Let's play a little game I like to call, "Instead of this, use that . . . "

Instead of expensive dumbbells use:

✓ Soup cans

✓ Bottles of water

✓ A jug filled with sand

✓ Socks full of coins

Instead of costly exercise equipment:

✓ Take a brisk walk or run

✓ Actually go rowing or kayaking

✓ Get on your bike and ride

✓ Walk up and down your steps

✓ Go roller skating

✓ Take a swim

Avoiding lactic acid

A common misconception is that lactic acid build-up is responsible for the muscle soreness and pain following a killer bout at the gym. Not so, my friend — the pain actually stems from the production and use of lactate in the muscle tissue. This pain is a protective mechanism, set in place to make you stop doing whatever it is you're doing before you permanently harm your muscle tissue.

Lactic acid is not evil, it's protective. If you've ever heard someone speaking of a recovery period (taking a day off) after strenuous exercise, it's because of this lactic acid build-up. Your body needs some time to decrease the inflammation and acid in your muscles. Muscles are composed of protein, and protein cannot function in an acidic environment. The pH of your muscles must recover and get balanced before protein can be used to build and repair them.

So, how do you avoid lactic acid build-up? By slowly immersing yourself in an exercise plan and making it a permanent part of your life. You always form acids from exercise, but your body becomes more efficient at removing them and you're less likely to permanently injure yourself if you go slow.

Getting started on an exercise plan

The very first step in starting any exercise program — whether you're a fitness maniac or just getting off the sofa — is to assess your current fitness level. This provides a starting point and a reality check. I'll never forget my first fitness assessment where I could do only five sit-ups and not even one push-up. Reality check, anyone?

If you have known medical problems or injuries, your doctor can help you assess your current level and develop a safe exercise plan, probably with the help of a physical therapist.

Checking your current fitness level

Before you get started, take a realistic look at your fitness level by answering a few questions.

Record your answers and set them aside. They'll provide a nice comparison in a few weeks when you reassess your fitness.

- ✔ How often do you exercise? (For how many minutes and how many days per week.) Experts agree that you should aim for at least 150 minutes weekly. That's about five, 30-minute sessions per week.

- ✔ What is your resting heart rate (RHR)? (A lower RHR may be indicative of better cardiovascular health.) A heart rate between 60 to 100 beats per minute is considered normal, although lower numbers (60 to 80) are more desirable because your heart isn't working as hard at rest.

✔ What is your Body Mass Index (BMI)? (A BMI of 18.5 to 24.9 is normal.) If it's higher than 24.9 you are considered overweight. Lower numbers may mean that you are too thin for your height.

✔ What are your circumferential measurements? (Chest, waist, and hips.) If your waist measures the same as your hips, you probably have an apple-shaped body, which is linked with a higher risk for developing cardiovascular disease. As opposed to a weight on your scale, watching your circumferential measurements get smaller with healthy diet and lifestyle changes are very rewarding!

✔ How long does it take you to walk one mile? The average adult can walk it in about 20 minutes at a leisurely three-mile per hour pace.

✔ How many sit-ups and push-ups can you complete in two minutes? Record these numbers for informational (and comparative) purposes only. There is no right or wrong number here, just a baseline of your callisthenic abilities!

✔ Complete a *talk test* during an exercise such as walking. Talk throughout the exercise and take note of how long you can go before you can no longer talk and work out at the same time. If you routinely exercise, the duration of your talk time should slowly increase.

Notice the absence of the "How much do you weigh?" question. Honestly, forget the scale — it's old school! Your answers to the other questions are much more indicative of your overall fitness level.

After you examine your current level of physical fitness, set some goals. Ask yourself what you hope to accomplish with exercise — a leaner, more toned body? Greater physical strength? Improved health? Keep your goals in mind daily, especially on those rainy mornings when you would rather have your eyelids surgically sewed shut than get on the treadmill.

Scheduling exercise

On average, an adult needs about 150 minutes of exercise weekly. You can divide up the time however you like, as long as you start slow and increase your exercise gradually.

There is no shame in scheduling a few ten-minute exercise sessions for your first week. Each week, as tolerated, tack on another ten minutes until you reach your daily exercise goal (preferably 30- to 60-minute sessions).

The best plan is to include a mix of aerobic workouts and two days of strength training (yes, I mean weight lifting) every week. I find that a 30-minute workout six days per week is good for me, and it provides 180 minutes of exercise per week! Table 6-1 shows my weekly plan.

Table 6-1		Sample Weekly Workout Plan				
Sunday	*Monday*	*Tuesday*	*Wednesday*	*Thursday*	*Friday*	*Saturday*
Rest	30 minutes aerobics or Zumba	30 minutes strength training (arms, back, and shoulders)	30 minute bicycle ride (no coasting)	30 minutes strength training (core, buttocks, and legs)	30 minutes Tai Chi	30 minutes Yoga

If you're just beginning an exercise program, repeat this mantra daily:

Go slow. Go steady. Let your body get ready.

Warming up and cooling down

Warm up and cool down before and after each exercise session. A good rule for the warm-up is to walk or jog in place and gently stretch the muscles you intend to use for about ten minutes. You want to increase your heart rate a little bit to prepare it for the increased oxygen demand you're about to make on it.

Similarly, a proper cool down lasts about ten minutes and includes gentle stretching while your muscles are still warm and limber. This time allows your heart rate and breathing to slowly return to normal.

Embracing cross-training

Just because I'm a nice person I'm sharing with you my best-kept exercise secret: mix it up. If you run five miles every day of the week, I'm happy for you, but I also know that you're not using all of your muscle groups. Worse yet, you're probably over-using your large muscle groups, keeping them in an acidic (non-protein using) state where they cannot build or repair themselves.

Experts recognize that *cross training,* or using different muscle sets every time you exercise, is important to being well-rounded physically. If you go rowing on Monday, give your arms, back, and shoulders a rest on Tuesday by scheduling a walk, jog, or run.

Reassessing your fitness

About six to eight weeks into your exercise program, it's a good idea (and a powerful motivator) to reassess your fitness level. Ask yourself the same questions posed in your initial fitness assessment (see "Checking your current fitness level" a bit earlier in this chapter) and record the answers. The first time I actually saw my BMI and measurements drop, I was hooked forever!

Acidifying Stimulants

This section will literally crack up anyone who knows me well. Once upon a time, I had a cup of coffee (sometimes multiple cups) in front of me at all times of the day. Hmm — go figure, my dieting and exercise efforts were going nowhere. I was acidifying my system with gallons of caffeine, and my body kept stuffing the acids into my fat cells to keep them away from my vital organs.

Your overly protective body goes one step further. After it has stowed away these acids in your fat, it actually decreases the circulation to said fat to prevent the acids from sneaking back out.

Again, these seem like little inconsequential choices — green tea or black tea, regular coffee or decaf — but they have a huge impact on your pH and overall health. When I learned I had to cut out my beloved 12 cups of coffee a day, I had to ask myself: If I don't want to jump into a pH balanced lifestyle with both feet and follow all the rules, am I ready to jump in at all? The answer was a resounding "yes," but I had to slowly wean off the caffeine, not just quit cold turkey. After getting my pH back on track, I found that giving myself a break and enjoying the occasional cup of java was better than quitting the diet altogether. Coffee is acid-forming, but the effects aren't cumulative if you take your treats in moderation.

Caffeine

I am *not* going to tell you to drop your coffee, tea, or caffeine source of choice. I am going to tell you how to improve the choices you make and how to work alongside your body (instead of against it) to decrease the acidifying effects of caffeinated stimulants.

As one of the main acid-forming stimulants, caffeine is one of the biggest culprits of acidity and pH imbalance. Think about how much caffeine you take in daily in the form of:

- Coffee
- Dark and milk chocolate
- Energy and performance drinks, bars, or pills
- Hot cocoa
- Soft drinks
- Tea
- Weight-loss pills

Mainlining caffeine may not be counterproductive to your health, although studies remain inconclusive (last week it was bad for you, this week it's okay). Even so, caffeine (and usually the vehicles it's carried in) are acid-forming, which is not good for your pH.

So even though one cup of coffee in the morning doesn't look that bad, it probably contains anywhere between 100 and 200 milligrams of caffeine, and the suggested upper limit is between 200 and 300 milligrams per day, depending on your size. Aside from acidifying you, all of this caffeine intake can also:

- ✔ Cause irregular heart beats
- ✔ Cause nausea
- ✔ Decrease your focus and concentration
- ✔ Interrupt your sleep and lead to insomnia
- ✔ Promote hyperactivity and irritability

If you're ready (and willing) to cut back on the caffeine, consider switching that black brew or soda for an alkalinizing cup of caffeine-free green tea or barley coffee. And here's a little side bonus: If you're a routine soda drinker, you may cut out as many as 1,400 calories a week by kicking the habit — that's equal to almost two pounds! Just imagine all the money I could make if there were a way to bottle that advice and sell it!

If you won't budge on the daily cup o' java (I feel your pain), consider drinking a large glass of lemon water before and after your brew. The alkalinizing water may help to combat the acidity of the coffee in your digestive system, and it will replace the fluids lost through *diuresis*. Coffee forces fluids out through your kidneys quicker than they are supposed to be flushed out, which is why you have to go to the bathroom shortly after drinking the stuff.

What's hiding in your soft drink?

Cola, soda pop, pop, soft drink — no matter what you call it, do you know what's in it? If I handed you a chilled can of artificial colors and flavors, additives, acidifiers, aspartame (or eight teaspoons of sugar), foaming agents, and preservatives, would you drink it? That may be just what you're doing every time you enjoy a cold soda.

Do we know what all these chemical additives do to your body? Evidence is mounting that more than a few of these sweet and yummy drinks (including the ones pulled from the shelves because their sweetener was a known carcinogen) can lead to anything from osteoporosis to cancer — is that a risk you're willing to take?

I don't blame you if you like the carbonated bubbles — they certainly are refreshing. The next time you reach for a soda, however, consider adding some fresh-squeezed lemon juice to your sparkling mineral water for an additive-free alkalinizing choice.

Tobacco

Cigarettes, snuff, stogies, pipes, hookahs . . . despite the myriad health warnings, we are still a society gripped by addiction to *nicotine,* the addictive chemical in tobacco. Tobacco products aren't only bad for your health (last I heard, they cause over a dozen different types of cancer), they're also pH wreckers.

Nicotine acidifies your body at the cellular level. Whether you smoke it or chew it, this chemical attacks every one of your cells and mutates them. This damage leads to inflammation and disease over time.

The chemicals in tobacco literally thicken your blood and make your heart, lungs, and entire body work harder than it should to circulate nutrients to your tissues.

Over time, tobacco use may lead to:

- ✔ Atherosclerosis (hardening of the arteries)
- ✔ Cancer
- ✔ Heart disease
- ✔ High cholesterol and blood pressure
- ✔ Lung disease
- ✔ Peripheral artery disease
- ✔ Stroke

In a nutshell, using tobacco is highly counterproductive to any dietary attempts to correct your pH. Think of it this way: Tobacco use is more acidifying than eating a side of beef, and the damage to your body is cumulative. The more tobacco you use, the more acids you stow away.

The bright light is that when you quit, your body immediately goes to work correcting your pH. Within about a year, your risk of heart disease and cancers drops to a more acceptable percentage (instead of being through the roof like it is now).

Getting the nicotine monkey off your back isn't easy in the least. Even though you consciously know it's bad for you (and now you know just *how* bad), it's still an addiction that takes a conscious effort to break — a continuous, conscious effort.

I've been coaching clients about smoking cessation on and off for years. The three main factors required to permanently quit include:

- ✔ **Support:** Unless you have some support , you won't succeed in giving nicotine the boot. If your family and friends aren't supportive, locate an online or local smoking cessation group and make new, positive friends.

> Limit the time you spend with former smoking buddies initially, as the temptation to light up or chew again is just too great.

✔ **Preparation:** Prepare for your quit date, which means setting one and sticking with it, by telling friends, cleaning out your home (if you smoke inside), and stocking up on hard candies, gum, or other, less-toxic substitutes. Get mentally ready and keep telling yourself that millions of people have quit before you — they aren't necessarily stronger than you, they were just determined.

✔ **Behavior modification:** This may sound like a new-wave parenting technique, but I assure you that's not what I mean. What I mean by behavior modification is to change the way you do things that led you to use tobacco in the first place and change the circumstances that are triggers for tobacco. For example, deal with stress by counting to ten, not by smoking. Try taking a walk after dinner instead of using tobacco.

Feeling Emotions Impact Your pH

Your emotions and mental health impact your pH. It's a proven fact that chronic stress has physiological impacts and can affect your health, response to medical treatment, and pervade every aspect of your life. Stopping stress from getting the best of you takes a conscious effort.

The two types of stress are:

✔ **Eustress** is a happy response to an exciting situation. Eustress may stem from a joyous occasion like an impending party, promotion, or successful business endeavor. It may also help give you the edge that you need to finish a large project or the mental clarity required to pass a test.

✔ **Distress** is the uncomfortable bodily response to tense, dangerous, or unfamiliar situations. It's the one that gives "stress" a bad rap.

Not all stress is bad, and not all stress harms your body. Check out Table 6-2 to learn the physiological differences between the good stress and the bad stress.

Table 6-2   Physiological Impacts Based on Type of Stress

Eustress (Good Stress)	Distress (Bad Stress)
Increases heart rate and blood pressure	Increases heart rate and blood pressure
Increases focus and concentration	Decreases concentration and retention
Excitement	Irritability
Gives a burst of energy	Leads to lethargy and exhaustion
Short-term only	Can be long- or short-term

Recognizing chronic stress signals

Chronic stress can eventually lead to illness or a disease process. At the least, chronic stress is the trigger for many uncomfortable symptoms including:

- ✔ Sleeping problems
- ✔ Gastrointestinal issues (nausea, diarrhea, gas, pain)
- ✔ Loss of appetite or over eating
- ✔ Irritability, anger, anxiety, and loss of concentration
- ✔ Headache (tension headaches or migraine triggers)

To add injury to insult, your body can actually get stuck in a chronic state of stress. It's almost like pushing down on the gas pedal and having it stick to the floorboard — you can't help it, but you are eventually going to career out of control or have a head-on collision. Understanding how to manage stressors — the bad ones — when they occur is the best way to resume control of your body's reactions.

Decreasing your stress response

You've probably seen the dozens of commercials promoting "happy pills" for stress or anxiety. Fact is, some people need pharmacological assistance, especially when chronic stress leads to depression (which I am not trained or qualified to talk about).

Most people can benefit from discovering how better to cope with daily stressors. The next time you find yourself in a stressful situation pay close attention to your responses, both physiological and emotional.

I got cut off in traffic this morning and had to slam on my brakes. My laptop and cell phone went flying off the front seat and had a meet-and-greet with my dash. Synchronously, several things happened:

- ✔ My heart rate sped up in anticipation of a traumatic event.
- ✔ My breathing increased to match the exertion of my heart.
- ✔ My muscles spontaneously contracted to help me get away from what I suspected was an impending collision.
- ✔ My pupils constricted to increase my visual acuity.
- ✔ My saliva and gastric secretions dried up. (Who needs those fluids in the middle of a car accident anyway?)

Collectively, this natural response to stress is part of your *fight or flight response* — yet another wonderful throwback from your caveman ancestry that helps your body prepare to either fight off an attack or run away from an overwhelming threat. Fact is, you can't stop this natural response from occurring — but you *can* recognize it and back down the severity of the response when it is unwarranted. If a cup of spilled coffee or a chipped nail are enough to set your teeth on edge, your fight or flight response may be stuck in the on position. The next sections offer various methods to help tone down your physiological and psychological barometers to reduce unnecessary wear and tear on your system.

Stress-reduction techniques can help an otherwise healthy individual decrease stress and defy the acidity associated with chronic stress. However, they are not a replacement for medical care. If self-help is not enough to dispel your stress, anxiety, or impending depression, please seek professional help.

Meditation

Hands down, meditation is one of the best methods you can use to reset your mind-body connection. *Meditation* is a purposeful mindfulness — you're giving your brain a break and looking at your situation from the outside (in a non-judgmental way). If you're stuck in high stress mode all the time, your body may need a healthy dose of relaxation.

Contrary to any stigma that remains, meditation is not some crazy alternative method to heal your body. You don't need soothing (or some would say spooky) music, candles, or even a white robe in order to mediate. However, some techniques can help you ease into meditation. You can get the basics on how to get started through a link to Stephan Bodian's *Meditation For Dummies* cheat sheet at www.dummies.com/how-to/content/meditation-for-dummies-cheat-sheet.html.

Neuropsychological studies prove that people who frequently meditate have healthier brain waves — how cool is that? Besides a cleaner brain, meditation may also:

- Improve your mood and make you happier
- Make you calmer
- Assist you in controlling stress or anger
- Physically relax you
- Help you connect spiritually with your Higher Power
- Improve your immune function

Have you ever sat at your computer or desk and zoned out? These moments of staring into space and concentrating on everything and nothing is meditation. You might've been meditating for years without knowing your action had a name. If you're up to the challenge, try doing it purposefully. Be sure to tell me how good you feel after!

Yoga

With yoga, you can take meditation one step further. *Yoga* is the marriage of meditation to specific postures called *asanas* and regulated breathing called *pranayama.*

Some of the benefits of a yoga practice include:

✔ Improved mood and relaxation

✔ Decreased stress and anxiety

✔ Increased flexibility and lung capacity (you breathe better)

✔ Decreased blood pressure and heart rate

I admit, the first time I tried yoga I felt more frustrated following the session than before I started (I am not a pretzel-like flexible person and I cursed more than I breathed). My suggestion? Find a personal trainer and start there. Practitioners of yoga can start you in a chair (chair yoga) and gradually ease you into some of the more high-speed yoga positions as you become ready.

There are many different types of yoga, which stem from their original country of origin. *Yoga For Dummies* by Georg Feuerstein and Larry Payne offers a variety of postures to try.

Guided imagery and deep breathing

You want a relaxation technique that's free and easy to learn and practice? Look no further than guided imagery and deep breathing.

Although the name *guided imagery* sounds highly technical, it's actually nothing more than conjuring up a pleasant vision and focusing on that image, as opposed to the stress or anger you may be feeling. The more details you put into your session (don't just imagine a beach — imagine a beach, sand on your toes, sun on your face, and seagulls cawing in the distance) the more you benefit.

Deep breathing is one physical way to stop your stress response in its tracks. When you start to feel stressed, your heart rate climbs. Purposefully take a nice deep breath and don't allow your body to go on hyperventilation overdrive. Personally, I like to count to five as I inhale and five as I exhale. Experiment with the combination that works for you and try it the next time you feel your heart rate or breathing pick up.

Find both of these techniques and more in *Relaxation For Dummies* by Shamash Alidina.

Balancing the Fluid Act

Plain water is essential to a healthy existence. Sure, you get fluids through coffee, soda, juice, and milk, but they don't contain pure water.

Your body has to exert energy (remember, energy exertion causes acid production) to separate molecules and extract the plain water from the other components in whatever you drink, such as soda or juice.

Water has a mind-blowing number of functions within your body. Unsurprisingly, up to three-quarters of your body weight is composed of water. Your brain is composed of mostly water as well, so a hydrated brain is a happy brain! Remember that hangover you suffered? It was due to an unhappy, dehydrated brain. Don't make your brain unhappy — it's the control system of your entire body. That's like poking the pilot of an airplane — big no-no!

Making your own sports drink

Most commercially manufactured sports drinks have the same claim to fame: They help you rehydrate and can help prevent dehydration during sports or exercise. The central rehydrating component of sports drinks is not a mystery — it's the essential electrolytes such as salt, potassium, and magnesium. When you start to exercise and sweat, these electrolytes pour out of your skin (hence the salt stains on your running clothes). Water goes where sodium flows — as your sodium (salt) flows out of your pores, your water follows it, and you run the risk of becoming dehydrated.

What most sports-drink commercials don't mention is the fact that one, eight-ounce serving of a commercial sports drink may have around 28 grams of sugar per serving (depending on the brand). Go get a teaspoon and eat seven spoonfuls of granulated sugar — it's the same thing as drinking 28 grams of sugar!

However, you can make your own sports drinks at home with almost half the calories

of the commercial brands (and honey rather than acidifying sugars). This formula is only for adults; use pediatrician-recommended brands for children. For a home-brewed electrolyte replacement system combine:

- 2 cups water
- Dash of fresh-squeezed lemon juice
- 1/4 teaspoon salt
- 3 teaspoons honey

I've heard of people also adding sugar-free lemonade mixes to make the drink more palatable but I like it as-is.

To avoid the nasty effects of dehydration (and to preclude the need to suffer ounces of oral re-hydration mix) be sure to drink water before, during, and after any kind of physical exertion — especially if it's warm outside.

Lubricating your body

Water acts as both lubricant and a source of moisture in your body. Just look at some of the tissues in your body that require water to function:

- ✔ **Eyeballs:** Your eyes are not only surrounded by water, they are full of the stuff. This is why you blink — to redistribute moisture over your oxygen-exposed eyeball.

- ✔ **Spine:** This sturdy muscular column is bathed in spinal fluids composed mainly of water. The spine also transmits signals via water, an electric conductor.

- ✔ **Joints:** You can bend your elbow, fingers, knees and wrists because water in synovial fluid surrounds the joint.

- ✔ **Bones:** Without this lubricant, you may start a fire by the friction of bone on bone while running . . . okay not really, but you see my point. (Yep, bones have water, too.)

- ✔ **Skin:** Your skin's elasticity is dependent on water. If you're not drinking enough, the top layer of cells appear dry, flaky, and wrinkled. (Do you have alligator skin? Could be you're not drinking enough water!)

Do a quick test to see how lubricated your skin is. Pinch the skin on the back of your non-dominant hand and release. Does the skin snap back into place, or does it stay tented in the pinched position? If the latter occurs, you may be dehydrated and don't have enough water to maintain your skin's elasticity!

Saliva (mostly water) acts as a lubricant to moisten and begin digestion of anything you put in your mouth. Just imagine trying to swallow if your mouth were as dry as the desert!

Transporting nutrients

Water is an amazing transportation vehicle. It helps you digest your food, transport nutrients, and even carries the garbage out. Your bodily fluids, including blood and gastric juices, are largely composed of . . . yep, you guessed it: water!

Your blood (all five liters of it) is water-based. It's the taxi service for nutrient transportation. The *circulatory system* is composed of a network of veins, arteries, and capillaries — it's the highway for nutrition distribution throughout your body. The arteries bring oxygenated, nutrient-rich blood to your tissues. The capillaries are the middlemen, where nutrients are exchanged at the cellular level. The depleted, oxygen-less blood is returned through your veins to your heart where it gets reoxygenated.

Gastric fluids and saliva break down nutrients so they can be absorbed at the cellular level. The salad I just ate needs to be broken down into its microscopic components before my body can make use of it.

Flushing out waste

In the form of urine, stool, and lymphatic fluids, water flushes waste and toxins out of your body. Once the nutrients are extracted from food, it becomes solid waste. This solid waste (stool) needs water to flow through your remaining colon to your rectum, where it's removed from the body.

Along with the solid and liquid waste, water carries acids out of your body (this is how urine pH testing illustrates your overall acidity, by showing the quantity of acids removed in your urine).

Water is probably the most important aspect of your acid alkaline diet. Water sweeps acids out of cells and is necessary for fat breakdown and removal. No water means no acid removal. It's no wonder you can't survive more than a few days without water!

Replenishing your body

Isn't it odd that the best thing you can do for your body is completely free? Depending on the quality of your local water supply, filtered tap water may be a perfectly acceptable exchange for the fancy plastic bottles of water (you'll also be doing a great thing for the Earth by using less plastic).

A good rule to maintain hydration is to drink half your body weight (in pounds) in ounces of water daily. If I weigh 120 pounds (uh-huh, sure), I should drink 60 ounces of water daily, or seven-and-a-half eight-ounce glasses. However, a 200-pound man obviously has more cells to hydrate and he needs more like 12.5 eight-ounce glasses per day! (Comparable metric measures: If you weigh about 54 kilograms, drink 1¾ liters of water a day; if you weigh close to 91 kilograms, drink close to 3 liters.)

Although I've heard arguments to the contrary, I believe that drinking water at room temperature is best. Your body easily absorbs room temperature water without any work. Drinking cold water makes your body expend energy heating the water to an absorbable temperature, and using energy means producing acid. So, try sipping tepid water.

If you need some help tolerating plain ole water, try adding fresh-squeezed lemon or lime juice to perk it up.

Chapter 7

Reversing Your Acidic Trend

· ·

In This Chapter

▶ Getting your body back on track

▶ Preparing yourself for a lifestyle change

▶ Debunking the myths about detoxifying and cleansing

▶ Setting reasonable expectations

▶ Understanding the impact of free radicals

▶ Avoiding common mistakes

· ·

*E*ven though it was intended for the business-minded, not the health con-scientious, I love Jack Welch's quote, "Change before you have to." This successful American businessman, who was acclaimed as manager of the century by *Fortune* magazine during his tenure as CEO for General Electric, succinctly stated the intent of this book in just five words. You can change your lifestyle, diet, and health for the better now or face the risk of having to change in the future, after disease has gotten a grip on your body.

Reversing years of acidity is not an overnight process, but it doesn't have to be fraught with despair and speed bumps. I show you how to avoid unsafe practices in pH balancing while setting realistic, obtainable goals for yourself.

This chapter presents important concepts that can help you turn an about-face to cellular damage. Once you understand the snowball effect going on in your body, you'll be ready to make better decisions for your health and well-being.

Altering Years of Acidity

Top four things you probably don't want to hear before starting this diet:

✔ Some diseases cannot be cured.

✔ Some damage may be irreparable.

✔ If it were easy, everyone would be doing it.

✔ Altering years of acidity takes time and effort.

In a society gripped by the "I want it now" mentality, that last one's a doozie and a turn-off for many people. I can't stand half-truths, which is why I'm putting this information out there. If you embrace the fact that a pH-balanced lifestyle is not a simple endeavor, you will be successful.

There are plenty of pH-balancing analogies to pull from, but my personal favorite uses the fish tank environment. Imagine that you have one fish living in a large tank. Also say that you go on vacation and forget to have Aunt Marge come baby-sit said fish. You return home to a green, slimy layer on the glass, cloudy water, and a fish seriously struggling to survive. You turn on the pump and start wiping the algae off of his glass. How long will it be until he is healthy and happy and the water is clear again? That depends on how dirty his water was, how good your filtration system is, and the overall health of your fish.

The point is: You are that fish. The amount of time required to reap the benefits of a healthy pH balancing lifestyle depends on how acidic your lifestyle was, how strong your body is, and your current level of health and well-being. It's also dependent on your level of commitment — if you just sort-of embrace the acid alkaline lifestyle, you may just sort-of get results.

Checking out your current health

I cover pre-existing medical conditions and talking to your doctor in Chapter 10 — but it's such an important topic that I want to hit on it here, as well. If you have a pre-existing medical condition, speak to your doctor before engaging in any dietary or lifestyle changes. Of course, I'm pretty sure your doctor will applaud if part of your lifestyle change is to quit smoking and start drinking more water!

For the rest of us who do not have pre-existing medical problems, cataloguing your current health can help you establish goals. You can't know how far you've come until you know where you started! (Is that a song verse?)

The easiest way to assess your general health (which should never take the place of a real medical examination) is by answering a few questions:

- When was the last time you were ill?
- How frequently do you get sick?
- What is your energy level?
- Do you have frequent digestive problems?
- Do you get headaches or feel tired frequently?

✔ Has your weight wildly fluctuated over the last few years?

✔ How many diets have you tried? How many diets have failed you?

✔ What does your doctor say about my health? Are you on track or have you received encouragement to diet, lose weight, or get better about scheduling routine screening exams?

When you're finished with the introspective inquisition, you're ready to take stock of your physical appearance. Are your hair, skin, and nails healthy and hydrated, or are they split, dull, and cracked? Are you pleased with your physical appearance, or do you hide behind loose-fitting clothing and elastic waistbands?

These and similar questions may provoke thought and a realistic assessment of your overall health and self-perception.

If you don't care for the answers, it may be time for a change in your diet and life.

Self-perception

If you're unhappy when you glance in that mirror, don't let it drag you down. According to theorists, your self-perception, or how you see yourself, is based on three things:

✔ What you see in the mirror

✔ What you think other people see

✔ What other people say they see

Although you cannot control what other people say or perceive, you can control your self-perception by focusing on the positive. It's a fact that constant negative talk can damage your self-image and confidence. It takes some time and effort, but your brain is the best tool in your self-image toolbox. The next time you feel a negative or self-depreciating thought coming on:

✔ Become your own cheerleader. List your positive attributes.

✔ Refocus your thoughts on how you plan to fix any perceived image problems, not just the fact that you don't like them. Don't say, "I hate my thighs," say "My thighs are going to look awesome."

✔ Listen to what others say, but don't bank on it. My mother always told me I was the most beautiful girl in the world. Of course it's nice to hear, but the opinion of other people should not define who you are.

✔ Pay close attention to your own thoughts. Do they tend to be negative? Incessant inner conversations like, "I shouldn't have eaten that cheesecake, I'm fat enough" or "I can't stand next to Tara, she makes me look like a whale" are going to kill your self esteem and perception. Pay attention to how you actually perceive yourself today, and start making a positive change in self-perception for tomorrow.

Setting realistic goals

You may not label them as such, but everyone sets goals daily. Masked as chores or daily responsibilities, these tasks are actually short-term goals. "Pick up the kids" and "buy milk" are well-defined immediate goals that you forget upon completion. Conversely, long-term goals like "finish my book" or "get my masters degree" require a little more thought and planning.

The acid alkaline diet and lifestyle require complementing short and long-term goals. I like to re-evaluate my life every so often and ask where I see myself in one year? Five years? Ten years? If you're drawing a blank, which I doubt, you can start thinking about your goals by asking yourself:

- What do I wish to accomplish with an acid alkaline lifestyle? Weight loss? Disease prevention? Put the brakes on my aging process?
- What is most important to me? How I feel or how I look?
- When I do expect to start seeing results?

The key word in this section is "realistic." If my goal is to be a 6'2" supermodel, all the planning in the world won't make this 5'8" mom star on the cover of Cosmo. The more realistic your goals are, the more attainable they are.

Putting pen to paper

Thinking about something and writing it down are two different concepts. If you think about it, the object remains intangible, dreamlike. Once you write down those magical words, you actually start your journey. It's like the match to a firecracker — you've set a chain of events in motion by taking the effort to write down your goals. Not convinced? Let me take that a step further.

Put your goals somewhere highly visible, like on the refrigerator door. The human short-term memory is very limited — it deletes any new information a couple seconds after it is learned. The only way to stop this process is by dropping your goals into your long-term memory files through repetition. Each time you walk by that fridge, you see your goals and they become solidified in your mind. That constant reminder is a powerful stimulus to make a change in your life!

Try to make each goal specific, timely and descriptive. Don't say, "I want to lose weight" because that is easily forgotten when the chocolate chip cookie dough ice cream cake makes an office appearance. Instead, consider writing something like, "I will lose five pounds by next month through dietary changes and exercise."

Examining your environment

Could your environment be contributing to acidity and poor health? Absolutely! One of my idols, Florence Nightingale, showed how a filthy environment breeds illness as far back as the 1850s in the Crimean War.

For this purpose, I define your *environment* as anything that you interact with externally, or outside of your body. The air you breathe, pollutants, and even your water supply are all part of your external environment. To a limited degree, you have some control over your external environment, thanks to science and human technology.

If your environment is ripe with pollutants and bacteria, your body is already working harder than it should to maintain health. Air pollutants can enter through your lungs (and skin), and bacteria can enter through your lungs, mouth, and skin. As your immune system fights to reject these environmental factors, your pH can suffer. Keeping a clean external environment reduces the workload on your immune system, which helps your body focus on the basics: Maintaining a healthy pH.

Maybe you cannot control where you live (big city versus rural farm), but you can control the germs inside your home or apartment. By nature, bacteria breeds an acidic environment. The more bacteria you take in, the more acidic your pH becomes. Some ways to reduce the pollutants within your home (and therefore create a healthier, less bacteria-breeding environment) include:

✔ Frequently change air filters, especially if you have pets.

✔ Use air purifiers if you are in a small space, such as an apartment.

✔ Take down (gasp) and wash your curtains or window treatments monthly.

✔ Wash bedding (including that comforter) weekly.

✔ Make sure your cleaning liquids read "sanitize" or "disinfect."

✔ Bleach your mop in between uses, or use disposable pads for floor washing.

✔ Frequently disinfect your electronics (think TV remote, phone, keyboard).

You can clean most electronic devices using a paper towel and disinfectant spray. Make sure you turn off the electronic device before attempting to clean it, and spray the paper towels, not the device. (I turn my laptop off before wiping down my keyboard so I don't accidentally blast off e mails!)

Although a pH-balanced body is more apt and able to fight these germs, why expose yourself if you don't have to?

Preparing for a New Life

Your body has the amazing capability of healing itself. This process starts the moment you stop bad habits! Quit smoking? Following that last cigarette, your body cleans up your lungs and blood within minutes. Within years, even your doctor may not be able to tell that you were once a smoker. Why? Because your body is busy healing itself behind the scenes, even more so once it no longer has to fight a constant acid bombardment. Given the opportunity, the human body can do some amazing stuff.

If you're only interested in starting an acid alkaline diet, you can skip to Chapter 9, where I show you how to start the diet. If you're ready to jump in with both feet and immerse yourself in a pH-balanced lifestyle, start preparing mentally as well as physically.

Getting mentally right

Your physical preparedness sets the stage for your mental transition into a new dietary lifestyle. Optimally, your goals are written out and hanging on the fridge (see "Putting pen to paper" earlier in the chapter), you've read up on how to start the acid alkaline diet (which I explain in Part III), and your exercise schedule is programmed into your smart phone (I cover the importance of exercise in Chapter 6). What now? Now that all of the physical tasks are complete, it's time to get mentally right and prepare for the task ahead.

 I'm a big fan of positive affirmations and self-talk. You're going to face challenges while transitioning to an alkaline lifestyle. Remind yourself (I do it while looking in the mirror) why you decided to embark on this journey in the first place. Something as simple as, "I can help my body achieve wellness" or as corny as, "I am the master of my own destiny" goes quite a way in bolstering your willpower.

Get in the right frame of mind by setting a start date and sticking with it. Avoid vague terms, such as "I'll start next week." Instead, pick a specific date to begin the acid alkaline diet and get your grocery shopping and meal planning done before that date.

You may find yourself going to the grocery store more frequently to restock your fruit and veggie supply on this diet. If you don't mentally prepare and make time for this minor inconvenience, it's easy to fall into old dietary habits and eat acid-forming side dishes, such as instant rice or potatoes.

 The single-most important piece of advice I can impart: Do not initiate change during times of duress. If you're planning a move, or a wedding, changing jobs, or doing anything that may cause stress and anxiety, wait until after the big event to get started.

Garnering support

Peer pressure is a powerful motivator. Some people choose to talk to family, loved ones, friends, and coworkers and tell them about your decisions *before* making a diet and lifestyle change. This method is frequently employed for long-time smokers or yo-yo dieters – peer pressure can be a powerful motivator! You may think twice about slipping up or quitting the diet once *every one* of your friends and family knows about it.

Acknowledging physical limitations

Acknowledging your physical limitations is the cornerstone of setting realistic expectations. I can face the truth — I'm never going to have the five-foot-tall perky body I've always envied because I'm shaped like a six-foot tree. Whether you're wheelchair bound, morbidly obese, or even a tree like me — incorporate your physical limitations into your expectations and embrace them.

The acid alkaline diet is not going to change your basic body type — no diet can do that. It can help you become a better version of you.

Forgiving mistakes

I've got to say it: You're not perfect. Neither am I, for that matter. I can predict with a high degree of certainty that you will make mistakes and fall back on old, comfortable habits while transitioning to a pH balanced lifestyle. How you react to those situations defines your capability of success (or not). The very first time you slip up and make a mistake:

- ✔ Forgive yourself.
- ✔ Pay attention to what triggered the mistake and avoid it in the future.
- ✔ Drink a glass of water and count to ten.
- ✔ Stow it away in your brain and don't nag yourself about it.

You can continue to use these same affirmations every time you slip up, with one consideration: If you're cheating on the diet daily, are you really on the diet? Sure, you can forgive yourself for eating that chocolate cake today, but if you turn around and eat it again tomorrow, you might want to give your willpower a boost by staying away from the source of temptation for a bit.

Making a mistake while dieting usually leads to one of two outcomes: quitting the diet or learning from the mistake. Take my advice and learn from your mistake — don't quit.

Cleansing Safely

Some people opt to complete an internal body cleansing — also known as a *detoxification* or *purification* — before starting the acid alkaline diet. The premise involves cleansing your body of as many toxins and acids as possible before starting the diet. Choosing to cleanse or not to cleanse is a highly personal decision that I cannot make for you.

I can tell you that a number of products claim to detoxify and don't. Some of them are even medically dangerous, so discuss any cleansing or detoxifying product with your health care practitioner before trying it. (Preferably even before buying it — your doctor may save you some money and tell you not to bother.)

Avoiding unsafe practices

Laxatives are composed of either natural or artificial chemicals that stimulate your body to release stool. Basically, laxatives force you to poop.

Sometimes laxatives are medically necessary, such as when you're constipated or before you're undergoing a screening exam of the digestive tract. However, there's no conclusive proof that sucking down ounces of laxatives will clean anything out of your digestive tract except for the fluid and electrolytes your body needs to survive.

Read the label on your cleansing or detox product before you buy it. A good practice of using supplements including knowing and understanding what you're putting into your body. Some common guises for hidden laxatives (both natural and manmade) include:

- ✔ Aloe vera
- ✔ Bran
- ✔ Buckthorn
- ✔ Castor oil
- ✔ Methylcellulose
- ✔ Psyllium husk
- ✔ Senna or senakot

You may be surprised to see bran, buckthorn, and aloe vera on this list, but I assure you that although natural, they are stimulants in the colon. I wouldn't be at all surprised if your "detox" or "gentle cleansing" supplement contains many plant parts, including leaves, berries, and roots. So I have to ask, "Do you need to pooh or are you paying money for a product claiming to do what your body already does?"

A cleansing detox is not intended for people who need to detox from drug or alcohol abuse. If you suffer from either (or both) of these addictions, seek help with a medical doctor and detox in a controlled environment, such as a rehab center or hospital. You may suffer seizures, hallucinations, heart problems, and much more unpleasantness while detoxifying from drugs and alcohol. Trying to detox from these substances at home is not only dangerous, it can be deadly.

Getting detox savvy

Don't assume any plant or herb is safe to take simply because you can purchase it without a prescription. Herbs are powerful, so talk to someone who knows what they're all about before starting to take them arbitrarily. Table 7-1 depicts some common detoxifying plants and how they're used.

Table 7-1 Dietary Supplements Used in Detoxification Blends

Herb	Part of Plant	Suggested Purpose
Aloe	Pulp and leaves	Soothe the gastrointestinal tract
Burdock	Root	Cleanse the blood
Dandelion (that yellow flowered weed in your yard)	Leaf and root	Improve liver, kidney, and digestive health
Fenugreek	Seed	May help decrease blood sugar and promote regularity
Ginger	Root	Increase gastrointestinal comfort
Juniper	Berry	Cleanse the kidneys
Milk thistle	Seed	Cleanse the liver, support liver cells
Parsley	Leaf	Cleanse the kidneys
Slippery elm	Bark	Cleanse the gastrointestinal tract

I am not an *herbalist* or *homeopathic physician* — medical professionals who are trained in the art of using herbs to improve wellness and combat disease. Any and all of these herbs may solicit side effects and interact with other supplements or prescription medications. Talk to your doctor before taking a herbal supplement.

I'm supposed to put the coffee where?!

An *enema* is a procedure in which liquid is inserted into the rectum via a plastic catheter to facilitate stool evacuation. Enemas are used to treat severe constipation or to cleanse out the colon prior to diagnostic procedures, such as a *colonoscopy* (endoscopic examination of the inner colon).

A disturbingly popular detoxification practice is the use of coffee enemas. Yep, this practice involves pumping your brew up your bum in hopes of cleansing the body and extracting toxins. Unfortunately, coffee enemas are gaining popularity as a whole body detoxification method. Supposedly the caffeine, when inserted directly into your rectum, helps to stimulate gall bladder, liver, and colon cleansing unlike the effects of simply drinking the stuff.

According to science, sticking a perfectly palatable ounce of coffee up your bum is not proven to do anything but waste java — although the caffeine is absorbed there as readily as it is in your tummy. Personally, if I feel like acidifying myself (caffeine is acid-forming) I will continue to sip the brew, not pipeline it into my rear.

Enemas, when inserted by non-professionals (whether they contain coffee or the more acceptable tap water), have the potential to cause *rectal perforations*, or holes in the walls of your rectum that must be surgically repaired. No thanks!

Years of scientific research have failed to prove that you can forcibly change the way your body removes toxins. Sure, you can speed up the gastrointestinal process (make yourself poo faster) — but does that really dump toxins at the cellular level? In my opinion, you already possess all the tools needed to detoxify your body: a pair of kidneys, a liver, and a colon.

Okay, now that I've trotted all over the concept of popular detoxifying products, let me tell you this: If you really want to clean out your colon and body, do it naturally. Drink more water (lemon water, if you please) and eat more fiber. Fiber is your natural broom — it sweeps all the yuck out of your colon, leaving only the good yuck (healthy bacteria) in place.

The natural fiber found in fruits and vegetables has benefits aside from cleansing; it fills you up. This satiety can result in weight loss and cholesterol reduction, plus it provides phytochemicals and enzymes that can only be found in a live product, not a pill. Overcooking fruits and veggies actually kills the good stuff like healthy chemicals and enzymes — so eat it raw and get maximum benefits.

Watching for false claims

In Canada, all natural health products, including detoxifying and cleansing products, must be approved by Health Canada and display a Natural Product Number (NPN) on the label. In order for a product to be approved, it must be proven safe and effective, and the manufacturers can only use justified claims on the package. Other countries similarly restrict and regulate dietary supplements. However, in the United States, most over-the-counter cleansing supplements aren't approved by anyone to do anything. Some of the claims aren't even valid — although those products usually get yanked from the shelves by the United States Food and Drug Administration. If the label claims are too good to be true, they most likely are! Beware of amazing claims such as:

- ✔ Lose 20 pounds in two days! (or the like)
- ✔ XYZ diseases cured!
- ✔ Order now, limited supplies!
- ✔ Absolutely no side effects!
- ✔ Totally safe!

This is by no means an all-inclusive list. Second-guess any cleansing supplement that promotes personal testimonials or fancy words — "purification of digestive flora" is a fancy way to say gets the bad germs out of your intestines — why didn't they just say that?

Your best bet when it comes to any cleansing or detoxifying product is to do your own research and talk to your doctor. Research yourself and check if the product is backed by a verifiable or trusted source (such as Health Canada or the United States Food and Drug Administration). Also look for:

- ✔ Contact information — can you reach a human being?
- ✔ Claims of side effects, known risks of taking the product

When in doubt, I'd avoid it. Your kidneys, liver, and colon work together with the lymphatic system to clean your body of all waste — you don't need to pay money to cleanse yourself, your body is already doing that (and will probably do it even better once you adhere to an acid alkaline diet and lifestyle).

Removing the Free Radicals

Nope, it's not a political group (although it does sound like one). *Free radicals* are actually biological trash, or the result of circulating garbage and debris from years of acidity, cellular damage, and waste stuck in your body. These atoms are electrically unstable, meaning they can target healthy cells and cause oxidative injury (which is why anti-oxidants are so vital to your existence and health).

It's argued that the build-up of free radicals over time is what leads to a natural human death. As you age, your body has a harder time removing this trash and difficulty keeping up with a constant influx of the stuff. The chronic build-up of free radicals is thought to increase your chances of developing chronic diseases such as:

- Cancer
- Autoimmune disease (where the body attacks itself)
- Premature aging

Free radicals are a natural byproduct of life — just as you have household garbage that builds up from living, your body has its own inner supply of garbage that builds up from sustaining life. But you wouldn't leave that household garbage in your home, would you?

Unveiling the free radical nemesis — antioxidants

The absolute nemesis to a free radical is the antioxidant. *Antioxidants* are kind and charitable compounds — they actually donate an electron to the free radicals that stabilizes them, which is coined as anti-oxidizing them. The neutralized free radicals are then removed safely from your body in urine and stool, without harming any further tissues on their way out. It's like subduing a violent criminal before taking him out of the club — if you knock him out, he will leave peaceful-like. If you don't, he may cause all kinds of damage before you move through the crowd.

Taking out the trash

So where do you find these peaceful antioxidants? In nature, of course! The compounds are hiding in fruits, vegetables, nuts, grains, and healthy proteins, such as fish and poultry. Your doctor may also encourage a daily multiple vitamin, which may provide a combination of antioxidants.

Vitamins A, C, E
It's no surprise that some of the most popular vitamins are also potent antioxidants. Vitamins A, C, and E circulate throughout your body and help neutralize free radicals and remove them — they take out the trash! Have you ever been told to take vitamin C for a head cold? The premise is that during this time, your body is busy fighting the virus that caused the cold and it may need extra help getting it out of your body.

Myth or method? The apple cider vinegar debate

Apple cider vinegar (ACV) is used as a weight-loss aid, gargle for sore throats, and even an astringent for dandruff. Although the scientific proof remains somewhat elusive, people continue to swear by this folk remedy. ACV lovers swear this tonic can also help remedy:

✔ Acne

✔ Diabetes

✔ Fatigue

✔ Flu

✔ High cholesterol

✔ Obesity

✔ Stomach disorders

The unpasteurized vinegar contains vitamins, minerals, and pectin — many of the healthful components of the whole apple itself. Cleansing practitioners may encourage drinking a diluted tonic of ACV to alkalinize the body. Although this vinegar contains acids, such as malic acid, they are quickly dissolved in your harsh gastric acids during digestion, leaving only the ash of minerals and vitamins (potassium, magnesium, beta carotene) behind.

Having said that, I don't think it's entirely safe to suck down vinegar, especially if you don't know what you're doing. ACV is an acid that can damage your tooth enamel and the soft tissues of your mouth and esophagus over time.

So, without drinking the stuff, what can you do with it? I've found that ACV works nicely for a random bout of dandruff. I used a solution of 50 percent water with 50 percent ACV. Applied to the scalp, it helped soothe the itching and cured my flakies. But take my word for this — don't get the stuff in your eyes. Ouch!

Eating a healthy, acid alkaline diet provides these anti-oxidizing vitamins in their natural form. In its natural form, vitamin A is found in animal products (so eat your salmon). Beta carotene, a precursor to vitamin A, is found in the colorful fruits and vegetables (carrots, strawberries, green leafies). Your body converts beta carotene into vitamin A in your small intestine.

Vitamin C is abundant in many fruits and vegetables, not just oranges (although they are a good source). Vitamin C hides in bell peppers, strawberries, and even tomatoes.

You may want to rethink your nutrition if you're getting the majority of your vitamin C from juice. Most juices have added sugars that are acid-forming, which negate the good of the vitamin C.

You're getting natural vitamin E if you eat nuts, seeds, and healthy oils. Vitamin E is also present in the dark green leafy veggies such as spinach and kale.

Beta carotene, lutein, and lycopene

Collectively, these compounds provide the fiery pigments in healthy plants (red, yellow, orange) and are called *carotenoids*. These potent antioxidants are absorbed in your small intestine and circulated throughout the body.

But there's a catch: Carotenoids need fat for proper absorption. I don't pair my fresh salads with avocadoes and olive oil just because it tastes good — the healthy fats in both avocadoes and cold-pressed olive oil help my body use the natural vitamins in my veggies! So pile on the carrots, tomatoes, and yellow peppers — these fiery fruits and vegetables provide a whopping dose of carotenoids.

Taking It Too Far

I'm not sure what percentage, but there is a percentage of readers who will try to rush results by forcing their body into an alkaline state. Yes, there are ways to do this, I just haven't talked about them because I don't think they're safe or right for everyone.

The only time there's a reason to rush your body into an alkaline state is during a medical emergency called metabolic or respiratory acidosis. These conditions of severe pH imbalance in your blood (your blood becomes acidic or is turning acidic with a pH less than 7.35) can ensue from:

- Diabetes
- Drug or salicylate (think aspirin) overdose
- Kidney failure
- Prolonged, untreated diarrhea
- Respiratory illness
- Shock
- Trauma to your chest

In all of these cases, medical treatment is required to rebalance your blood pH and monitor your condition closely.

If you try to force your pH balance to shift with pills and potions, you run the risk of taking it too far (hence creating a medical emergency where you become too alkaline — yes, this is possible). However, it is virtually impossible to become too alkaline by eating a healthy alkaline-forming diet, no matter how much salad you eat in one sitting. Chances are, you would vomit before you overdosed on alkaline-forming foods.

Avoiding common mistakes

I provide instruction on measuring your urine or saliva pH balance in Chapter 4 to help guide you through your acid alkaline journey, not to make you obsess over readings. A common pH-balancing mistake occurs when people start to ponder their pH levels and read too much into a simple urine test.

Avoiding overcompensation

Overcompensating for an acidic pH can have disastrous results. Like I said, it is possible to make your body more alkaline with over-the-counter supplements containing minerals, but it's not recommended. Supplements that may lead to overcompensation for acidity include:

- Alka-Seltzer
- Maalox
- Milk of magnesia
- Mylanta
- Rolaids
- TUMS

Do you see the trend here? All of these drugs neutralize acid (stomach acid, specifically). You need acid — just not nearly as much as you're probably getting in your current diet if you eat the Standard American Diet (SAD).

Speak to your doctor if you take potassium-wasting diuretics, as these drugs also have the potential to put your body in an extremely alkaline state and you may need to go slow while starting an acid alkaline diet.

Keeping an eye on the food pyramid

Eating an alkaline-based diet doesn't mean you should toss food groups and dietary recommendations out of the window. Actually, I think you should reconsider any diet that says you shouldn't eat a specific food group! The five main food groups are

- Dairy
- Fats and oils
- Fruits and vegetables
- Grains
- Protein

Check out the recipes in Part IV. I include a little of each food group in these recipes. A healthy, well-balanced diet doesn't cut out an entire food group! You need a variety of foods from each group to meet your body's needs.

Watching out for Internet scams

Anyone who hops onto the Internet can find hundreds of proprietors selling alkalinizing products. Just because you can buy these pills, potions, and kitchen gadgets, does that mean you should?

You're reading about the acid alkaline diet online one night and find what you hope is reliable information. Or is it? It's prudent to check the source before you start reading — what does the author have to gain by writing this blog or article? Is it merely knowledge dissemination or is there a hyperlink somewhere telling you to buy their alkaline products? Your first warning sign should be the myriad products and testimonials wallpapering the site.

If you go online intending to make a purchase, make sure you research the seller thoroughly before buying any alkalinizing product. Check the site and see if you can find:

✔ How long the seller has been in business

✔ A phone number or physical address (not a PO box) for returns

✔ A cancellation and returns policy (not a money-back guarantee only)

✔ Links to any peer-reviewed studies about the product

I always tell my patients to look for "dot-org, dot-edu, or dot-gov" when I teach them how to look up reliable information on the Internet. Usually, these HTTP suffixes denote an official or a not-for-profit site, where you're likely to find reputable, verifiable information. They may look like this: `http://www.my example.`**org**, `http://www.myexample.`**edu**, or `http://myexample.`**gov**.

Chapter 8

Getting Personal about Your Plan

*I*f you've tried and failed diets in the past, you already know how disheartening it is. But wait — there's still time to change (sounds like a TV ad, doesn't it?). Your body continues to heal and renew itself throughout your entire life, producing billions of new cells daily. Your hair, nails, and skin physically demonstrate this growth and renewal — and it's happening on the inside, too.

Are some people naturally more acidic than others? Probably, but your genetic make-up is not the only factor influencing your innate acidity. This chapter helps you to be honest with yourself — are you a meat-aholic? Type A personality? Emotional eater? You can't address the problems causing your natural tendency towards acidity until you admit to them.

Personally, I was shocked to learn that I was eating about 500 more calories daily than I needed. Understanding your body's true calorie requirements is an important aspect of eating right and regaining your health. You can eat a fairly strict acid alkaline diet and still suffer weight problems until you understand your body's basic energy requirements.

If you've read any other section in this book, you already know I'm big on taking baby steps. I fully believe it's the only way to implement permanent change. When you embrace past failures and examine them, you're stepping onto the path of personal growth and making the acid alkaline diet a part of your life.

Assessing Your Natural Tendencies

While counting down the days until your diet starting date, consider your natural tendencies that conflict with an acid alkaline diet and lifestyle. Natural tendencies are things you are predisposed to. You don't have to keep eating tons of beef; it's just what you've always done.

You cannot change your *deoxyribonucleic acid* — your DNA. Your DNA is your genetic fingerprint. It tells your body where and how to store fat, what color your eyes are, and even modulates your personality to a degree. (When was the last time your partner said, "You're acting just like your mother!")

I don't know of any genetic tendency towards acidity. Your body programs the amount of eggs you have in your ovaries (ladies) and the amount of fat cells you have in your body, but it doesn't program how many acids you dump into your system. That's like saying I can control the weather tomorrow!

I often see tendencies towards acidity reflected in the statements people proclaim about themselves:

- ✔ "I can't help it I have a sweet tooth."
- ✔ "I work full time — I don't have time to exercise."
- ✔ "A glass of wine helps calm me down."
- ✔ "I don't quit smoking because I don't want to."

Excuses, excuses, excuses. These statements reflect a lack of willpower and ability to control natural tendencies.

The following sections help you explore your personal tendencies to expose your Achilles' heel. Fight weakness by understanding it, facing it, and changing it.

Logging your pre-diet pH

If you read Chapter 4 and have your pH strips ready, you can start logging your pH and nutrition choices prior to starting the acid alkaline diet. I don't want to turn your acid alkaline journey into a chemistry experiment, but I think understanding your baseline pH, or your pH prior to any manipulative efforts, provides a nice starting point.

Consider giving yourself at least one full week of readings if you're going to track baseline pH. A day or two of pH results isn't truly reflective of your natural pH — it's probably reflective of whatever you ate and how much you exercised over the last two days. Be honest with your diet and your measurements while you're recording a baseline. What I mean is, don't eat better simply because you want your readings to look more alkaline. You should be seeing that soon enough.

Do mosquitoes love you?

I'm one of those people that attracts every mosquito within a ten-mile radius. While my friends and family sit on chaise lounges and enjoy the warm summer evening, I'm busy swatting and growing itchy red welts. Well, it turns out that there is a scientific reason for my suffering.

Mosquitoes have an incredible sense of smell, and they're choosy little biters. The female mosquito (males don't bite) picks her victim out of the crowd based on the way they smell. Mosquitoes actually show preference and prefer people who

✔ Are warm

✔ Breath out large volumes of carbon dioxide (the faster you breathe, the more you blow out)

✔ Pregnant (oops, no I'm not)

✔ Sweat (they love the lactic acid on your skin)

Although it's flattering to know that these pests like my personal bouquet, I'm not delighted about the fact that they transmit diseases like West Nile and malaria. These pests have survived hundreds of millions of years on instinct and their adaptability to change. They know that a cow tastes better than a tree, which is why plant-based pest repellants work so well. No self-respecting mosquito would bite a tree! Until science finds a way to mask our smelly mosquito-attracting compounds, keep yourself protected with a safe repellant.

Uncovering your acidic nature

You may tend to be more acidic depending on your personality type, geographical location, and even your culture. You may be thinking, "So what? I'm not going to relocate and I certainly can't change my personality." This is all well and true, but the fact remains: You can't address your weakness until you find it. Depending on your location, some acid-forming tendencies may be more culturally acceptable or even encouraged — think Americans and smoking or the French and drinking wine. Your cultural background also shapes the way you were taught to eat. Whereas I was raised on beef and potatoes, a friend from Spain grew up eating chorizo and rice. Both are examples of acid-forming diets that we've learned to enjoy through culture and family.

Although my psychologist buddies are sure to tell me it's antiquated, I still classify people by the ABC personality type theory started by Jacob Goldsmith. The three personality type descriptions include:

✔ **Type A:** Ambitious, truthful, impatient, workaholic, and quick to anger

✔ **Type B:** Easy going, poorly organized, apathetic, and sensitive

✔ **Type C:** Emotionally suppressed with poor or no coping mechanisms

I can clearly find myself on that list. Can you? Some people have cookie-cutter personality traits of a solid Type A or B, whereas others have a blend of two or more.

It's probably no surprise that Type A people tend to be more acidic. Type A folks worry, stress, and micromanage themselves, which results in excess acidity. Having said that, Type A folks also have one shining advantage: When they set themselves to a task, they stick with it!

The relationship between Type B and C personalities and acid proclivity is not as clear. I could hypothesize that due to their easy going natures, Type B people tend to carry less stress and therefore produce less acids than Type A folks. Conversely, Type C folks, who have limited coping skills, may overreact to a straightforward situation and increase their acids from stress. Regardless of your personality type, I suggest reviewing some of the relaxation techniques stuffed into Chapter 6. A couple minutes of meditation, yoga, or deep breathing can help you no matter what your personality type.

You may not be able to alter your intrinsic personality type, but you can alter your external responses.

Admitting you're a meat addict

Your success on a largely plant-based diet may depend on your level of affinity to meat and animal products. Honestly, just how carnivorous are you? Taking a realistic look at your current level of animal product consumption may help you understand how much your diet needs to change. Use the enlightening quiz in Table 8-1 to reveal if you're a meat addict.

Table 8-1	How Carnivorous Are You?		
Statement:		*True*	*False*
I eat meat or dairy as a part of every meal.			
I frequently use butter and cheese in cooking.			
Meat and dairy are the staples of my diet.			
Meat is my only source of B vitamins and iron.			
I enjoy hot dogs and luncheon meats four or more times per week.			

If the True column is filled, you may have a wee bit of a meat addiction. Meat is not the only source of vitamin B and iron, although that is the argument most meat-eaters use. Dark green veggies (such as spinach), grains, lentils, and fortified soy products also provide these nutrients.

It's okay if you filled the True column; now that you're aware of your tendencies, you can address them.

Although they are a good source of protein, vitamins, and minerals, animal products shouldn't take center stage on your plate in a pH balanced diet. You can get most of the same nutrients from plant foods:

✔ Grains, fortified soy products, dark green vegetables, walnuts, and lentils provide the zinc, vitamin B, iron, and omega 3 fatty acids found in meat.

✔ Tofu, soy yogurt, enriched soy or rice milk, and dark green vegetables provide the calcium and vitamin D found in milk and other dairy products.

If you're getting nervous about starting the acid alkaline diet, take a few minutes to peruse through the variety of recipes I provide in Part IV. Are you surprised to see a sprinkling of meat here and there? As long as the majority of your intake is alkaline-forming, there's no harm in still having a little animal flesh sparingly.

Cross-Examining Past Failures

Sometimes it's much easier to rationalize failure than to actually address the cause. If you admit that you failed your last diet due to (insert reason here), you're less likely to repeat that mistake. A coworker of mine was complaining about being overweight and attributed her problem to a "slow metabolism." She wasn't too happy when I brought up the meat-lover's pizza she ate for lunch.

It's human to fail. Examining the reason behind failure is how you grow, learn, and change. If you want to be successful on a pH balanced diet, think about past dieting attempts, types, and why you ultimately quit. Consider:

✔ Did the diet make you eliminate entire food groups?

✔ Did you starve or severely restrict calories?

✔ Were your taste buds bored?

✔ Was the diet expensive or technically challenging to adhere to?

In some of these cases, the diet actually failed you, not the other way around. An acid alkaline diet doesn't eliminate food groups and should not be boring.

If you've started the diet and feel that it's growing tedious, perhaps you aren't enjoying the variety of nature's bounty? Think about mixing it up by experimenting with new recipes, tastes, and textures. If you're an iceberg lettuce, carrot sticks, and chicken man, it may be time to toss in some strawberries, broccoli, and steamed salmon.

Conceding there's room to learn

If you don't know, you can't do. Sounds convoluted, but it's a fact that you can't embark on a diet if you don't understand the ins and outs of it. Some of today's dieting trends are so intricate and scientific that you practically need a Ph.D. to figure them out (or a calculator, at the least). I don't know about you, but I don't have that much time to dedicate to my food, and I know I wouldn't stick with a diet with complicated combinations or calculations. If I'm counting anything throughout the day, it's the number of minutes until I can go home from work, not the ounces, calories, and net calories that I just ate.

Living an acid alkaline diet requires one tool: your brain. Understanding the difference between acid- and alkaline-forming foods and the impact of pH on your body is all the knowledge you need to get started.

Taking baby steps

Astronaut Neil Armstrong said it best: "That's one small step for man, one giant leap for mankind." The best way to approach any change in your life — drastic or otherwise — is through small steps. Change isn't a tangible process; it's fluid and untouchable. Take baby steps toward your goals, and you have a better chance of making it to the finish line.

Chances are, you're already doing some things right. Do you take walks? Eat some vegetables? The trick is improving and building upon the good things you're already doing. Even if you only eat canned green beans once a week — it's a start. Tomorrow, think about switching those canned beans for the fresh kind. Next week, add some salad one day. See my devious plan unveiling?

Don't forget to pat yourself on the back along the way. Celebrate success — positive reinforcement is a powerful tool. Indulge in something that makes you happy, like taking an hour of solitude at the spa or having a movie night out with your partner.

Calculating Your Caloric Needs

Calories, or the measurement of a food's energy potential, carry the same stigma in today's society as a used bandage at a water park. They're seen as horrible, nasty little things that must be avoided at all costs. The fact is, calories are not horrible — they're necessary to survive. Eating calorie-dense, non-nutritive foods . . . now *that's* horrible.

Are you a pear or an apple?

Yeah, I'm not a piece of fruit either, but I'm talking about your body shape. Superimpose an apple or a pear over your body and see what one is closer to your shape. "Apples" tend to have larger waistlines and smaller buttocks, whereas "pears" have a small waistline with generous hips and buttocks.

Medical science acknowledges that the shape of your body predisposes you to chronic illnesses such as diabetes and heart disease. If you're an apple, you have about a three to five times increased risk of developing these diseases at some point in your life, as opposed to your pear-shaped buddies.

In truth, apples are more likely to develop *metabolic syndrome,* which is a collection of specific risk factors for heart disease and diabetes. Researchers have discovered links between metabolic syndrome and obesity, or being morbidly overweight, and a sedentary lifestyle. There's a chance you have metabolic syndrome if you have an apple shaped body and any three of the following:

- ✔ High blood pressure (either the top or the bottom number)

- ✔ Elevated blood sugars

- ✔ Too little good cholesterol (HDL)

- ✔ Increased fats (triglycerides) in the blood

- ✔ Waist measuring greater than 35 inches for women, 40 inches for men

If you are (or could become) an apple, take care to watch your diet, activity level, and waistline to avoid developing metabolic syndrome and its associated risks.

You can save yourself hundreds of dollars on prepackaged meal and diet plans by considering these caloric facts:

- ✔ To keep your weight stable, the number of calories you eat must equal the energy you put out.

- ✔ To lose weight, the number of calories you eat must be less than the energy you put out.

- ✔ To gain weight, the number of calories you eat must be more than the energy you put out.

Your body burns a given number of calories daily just to sustain life, which is known as your *basal metabolic rate* or BMR (some professionals also refer to it as the *resting metabolic rate* or RMR — same thing, different name). Your BMR won't be the same as mine; it's measured using your body weight, height, gender, age, and lean muscle mass (people with more muscles burn more calories).

Figuring out your body fat

To calculate your BMR, you need to know your percentage of body fat. You can do this in a number of ways:

- **Skin fold measurement (caliper test)** uses a small, painless tool, a caliper, to measure the thickness of your skin folds. The measurements are taken at several sites (underarm, hip, waist). Because the majority of your fat lies under your skin, this method loosely correlates your body fat percentage with the size of your skin fold measurements.

   You can get caliper testing done by a physical therapist, personal trainer, or anyone trained to administer the test.

- **Submersion test (hydrostatic tank measurement)** is also known as the dunk or water test. You are submersed in a large tank to obtain the "true" weight of your bones, muscles, and organs. Body fat floats, so the submersed weight is then compared with the dry weight, providing an accurate reflection of your weight in fat versus your weight in lean body mass. Submersion tests are available at some universities and physiology laboratories.

- **Bioelectrical impedance test** uses the premise that electricity travels slowly through fat and other dense tissues, but travels rapidly through tissues full of water, such as muscles. This harmless electrical current then sends feedback to a tiny computer to determine how much of your weight is composed of fat. You can find specialized bioelectrical impedance scales at medical equipment suppliers, but they are costly and somewhat unreliable (test results may vary depending on your hydration status). A trainer or physiological lab may complete bioelectrical impedance testing.

- **Dual Energy X-ray Absorptiometry scan (DEXA)** is a medically prescribed test; you cannot get a DEXA scan without your doctor's order. This painless test uses a radiographic scanner to differentiate between soft tissues and bone, and is primarily used to measure bone density.

   If your insurance does not cover the scan, it can be costly. DEXA scans, although the most accurate way to measure body fat, are not the most economical choice for the average adult. They are performed at hospitals and outpatient clinics. Talk to your healthcare provider if you are interested in having a DEXA scan.

You can also get a rough (very rough) guesstimate by some body-type comparison. If you're female and look

- Like a bodybuilder, your body fat may be around 9 or 10 percent
- Like a toned athlete, your body fat may be around 12 to 15 percent
- Like a Victoria's Secret model, you're looking at 18 to 20 percent

> ✔ Slightly overweight, you may have 25 percent body fat
>
> ✔ Definitely overweight, you may have up to (and more than) 30 percent fat

Men don't have the same fat reserves that females bodies hoard for procreation, therefore they have lower body fat percentages naturally. If you're a male who

> ✔ Looks like a bodybuilder, your body fat may be between 5 and 8 percent
>
> ✔ Has the look of an athlete, your body fat may be between 9 and 11 percent
>
> ✔ Is a muscular guy but without definition, you're looking at 12 to 16 percent
>
> ✔ Is slightly overweight, you may have 20 percent body fat
>
> ✔ Is overweight, you may have 25 percent or more body fat

Feeding your lean body mass

After you know (or have estimated) your body fat percentage, you are ready to figure out what part of your body weight is composed of lean muscles, organs, and bones.

To find your lean body mass:

1. **Multiply your weight in pounds by your percent of body fat.**

   The equation for a 120-pound woman with 16 percent body fat looks like: $120 \times .16 = 19.2$.

2. **Subtract that answer from your total weight.**

   Continuing the example: $120 - 19.2 = 100.8$

Lean body mass is the measurement of your body's *essential weight,* which includes muscles, tissues, and bones — the weight of the parts you need to survive. Exercise physiologists and trainers use this lean body mass to properly calculate how many calories you should eat daily to gain, stabilize, or lose weight.

The calories you eat daily provide energy for your lean body mass; if you eat too many calories, the extra calories turn into more fat.

Your BMR does not take pounds of fat into account — fat sits idle and doesn't need, use, or burn calories.

Understanding your BMR

If you know how much lean body mass you have, you're ready to calculate your BMR! Your *BMR* is the number of calories you need to consume daily just to survive.

You can use a couple of different formulas to calculate BMR (you can find a number of them online for free).

Personally, I like the Katch-McArdle formula. It's a simple and fairly accurate assessment of daily caloric requirement. Man or woman, to find your BMR using this formula, follow these steps:

1. **Convert your pounds of lean body mass into kilograms by dividing the number by 2.2.**

   Taking the 120-pound model with the 16 percent body fat (don't you just hate her?) with 100.8 pounds of lean body mass, the formula looks like this:

   $100.8 \div 2.2 = 45.8$ kilograms of lean body mass

2. **Multiply the result from Step 1 by 21.6.**

   So, $45.8 \times 21.6 = 989.28$, which you can round to 989.

3. **Add 370 to the result.**

   Add $989 + 370 = 1{,}359$.

   So, the sample model needs 1,359 calories daily just to sustain her life-giving functions.

This calculation does not include her five-mile run this morning or the fact that she works standing on her feet for 12 hours a day. The more you expend energy — whether at work, play, or exercise — the more calories you need to eat to fuel your body. If you want to know more about exercise and calories burned, check out the upcoming section, "Adjusting intake to your activity levels."

If you hate math or don't own a calculator, I'll give you a quick way to eyeball your BMR — just know that it's not entirely accurate. Multiply your weight in pounds by 15. The resulting number represents an estimate of your daily caloric requirements, but it doesn't take your lean muscle mass, height, or fat into account.

Adjusting intake to activity levels

The term *active* may mean something completely different to you than it does to me. Your activity level factors into how many calories you need to eat every day. If your daily activity consists of pressing buttons on the television's remote control for 12 hours, you probably don't need to eat much more than your BMR requirements, which I help you estimate in the preceding section. However if you work out, have active children, and spend zero time on the couch, you're going to burn more calories throughout the day.

Because most people like to overestimate their activity level, I've included loose definitions of the levels and how to adjust your caloric intake accordingly:

- **Sedentary:** You don't have a physically demanding job, and you don't routinely engage in exercise or physical activities. (It may even be a chore to walk over and pick up the TV remote.)

  To maintain your bodyweight, aim to eat your BMR requirements only.

- **Active:** You may be the taxi service for your kids and work a desk job, but you get moderate exercise at least three or four days each week.

  You need to eat the extra amount of calories that you burn each day to maintain your bodyweight. If you run on the treadmill for 45 minutes and burn 150 calories, you need to eat an extra 150 calories or you'll start to lose weight by burning body fat for that additional energy requirement.

- **Very active:** You either have a very physically demanding job (like heavy construction), or you're a gym fanatic. You work out vigorously at least five days per week and make sure you log more than 150 minutes of exercise weekly.

  Your body is burning large amounts of calories that need replenishing to maintain your bodyweight and your lean muscle mass.

How much do you exercise?

I would love to say that I exercise "vigorously" during the week, but when looking at the true descriptions, I'm more of an active kind of person. Ranging from sedentary (couch potato) to vigorous, your weekly activity level is measured by how much you move during the day. If you have a desk job but schedule time for workouts, you are probably still an active person. If you're retired and walk the dog once a week, you are technically a sedentary, or non-active person. See if you can match the activity level with the right description. The answers are provided at the end of this sidebar.

1. Sheila has a desk job but exercises two or three times a week.

2. Paul is retired and exercises maybe once a week.

3. Julia exercises at least four times weekly and works as a sales associate.

4. Juan does not schedule exercise, but he works six days a week in construction.

5. Marion works full time as a nurse and exercises at least three times a week.

Answers: 1. Light activity, 2. Sedentary, 3. Moderately active, 4. Vigorous, 5. Active

Taming your metabolism

The word *metabolism* is a fancy word describing how fast your body burns calories. It's also a common crutch used by healthy people who are overweight (I say "healthy" because there are some people with true metabolism disorders that affect their ability to lose weight, but it's not common). "I have a slow metabolism," and "My metabolism shut down when I hit 40," are common statements I hear, but they're not technically accurate.

I've heard only of two scientifically proven methods to boost your metabolism:

- ✔ **Eat routinely.** When you starve yourself, your metabolism slows down to conserve calories and energy. (It's a protection mechanism from your caveman ancestors).

- ✔ **Exercise.** Making your body exercise routinely is like hitting the gas pedal in your car. The body becomes a more efficient fuel-burning machine over time and your metabolism revs up.

Conversely, if you don't exercise and you frequently skip meals, your metabolism will slow itself — it's not some cosmic occurrence or your aging that's doing it.

Your metabolism and pH are directly linked at the cellular level. A chronically acidic pH inhibits your body's use of protein, which means you can't build or repair muscle tissue, and you may use energy less efficiently. If you want a faster metabolism, your best bet is to keep those cells less acidic, eat healthy meals (no skipping breakfast!) and exercise.

Part III
Making the Switch: Starting Your Diet

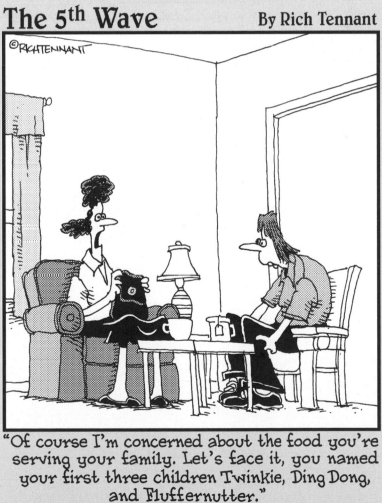

The 5th Wave   By Rich Tennant

©RICHTENNANT

"Of course I'm concerned about the food you're serving your family. Let's face it, you named your first three children Twinkie, Ding Dong, and Fluffernutter."

In this part...

It's time to dig into the deep, dark recesses of your pantry and refrigerator. Many acid-forming foods are hiding on your shelves — the staples of the acid alkaline diet are rarely found in boxes or prepackaged products. Reading over lists of acid and alkaline forming foods only gets you so far, but I provide them for a rough guideline.

The following chapters help you prepare to begin your pH journey by illustrating why certain foods and their ingredients are acid-forming. This way, you can make good food choices even if you leave your acid alkaline food list at home.

If you have any kind of chronic medical condition, I encourage you to consult your doctor before starting any diet or exercise plan. A pH diet is a healthy choice for most adults, but you may need to tweak it a bit.

Chapter 9

Checking Out Your Cupboards

. . . .

In This Chapter

▶ Considering what you eat

▶ Overcoming the excuses

▶ Cutting the costs

▶ Getting your family to eat right (and cut their acids, too!)

. . . .

*W*hen was the last time you really took a good, hard look at what's hiding in your cupboards? Some of my close friends have lived in the same house for decades, and you'd shiver if you heard what was hiding in the back of their pantry. (I won't even talk about their freezer because they would disown me.) Box of hamburger mix from 1992 — check. Canned peaches in heavy syrup from 1994 — check. Even if you live in a hurricane or flood zone (and hence may need the army-sized supply of food in case of an emergency), it's good practice to rotate your nonperishables and take a peek at the dates every few years!

This chapter is going to help you clear your pantry, freezer, and fridge of the acidifying yuck that most of us live on. In fact, the majority of your dietary acids are probably hiding on your shelves. I just have to say it: How many preservatives do you think hide in a can of food that can live on the shelf for ten years? It's time to dust off those cans and restock your fridge and pantry with acid alkaline diet staples. I'll even give you some money-saving tips while doing so.

Excuse-makers beware — this chapter covers all the excuses people use to continue eating that processed garbage. I used to do it (rationalize bad food choices) so I'm pretty much a self-proclaimed expert on the subject.

Cleaning Out Your Pantry (and Fridge and Freezer)

Cleaning out your fridge, freezer, and pantry has a two-fold purpose:

✔ For starters, it makes you take a hard look at what you eat on a day-to-day basis. If your refrigerator's produce bin is stuffed with processed lunch meats and the door is overflowing with bottled condiments, it's no longer an "ice box," it's an "acidity box."

When you start filling the fridge with fresh fruits and vegetables, and start using the freezer to hold pre-prepared healthy meals, you're well on your way to an alkaline diet and lifestyle.

✔ The more devious part of this cleaning plan is to make you toss acid-forming foods — you can't eat what's not there. Next time you're hungry and the microwavable mac-n-cheese is no longer in your pantry you'll thank me.

After you get rid of all the acid-forming foods in your pantry, fridge, and freezer, you may be wondering what the heck you're going to make for dinner. Skip ahead to "Getting your staples" for a grocery list. You can pick any of the healthy recipes in Chapters 14 through 17 and make them using some of the ingredients on that list.

Keeping natural disaster provisions

I've put up hurricane shutters in gale-force winds, survived an earthquake in San Francisco, and read about horrendous destruction following tornados and mudslides across the globe. If you live in a region subject to natural disasters, it's prudent to keep at least a three-day supply of provisions in your pantry. (Personally, we keep a week's worth.) Consider stocking:

✔ Baby formula (if you have an infant)

✔ Bottled water and sugar-free juices

✔ Canned fruit and vegetables

✔ Canned low-sodium tuna fish or salmon

✔ Granola and nuts

Don't forget to have a can opener handy as well as packing a supply of any prescription medications you or a family member requires. Better yet, know the evacuation route for your region, and have a family emergency plan ready.

Peeking in your pantry

I bet that over half of your cupboard contents are acid-forming foods — because most of these foods are convenient and have a shelf life of decades. I'm not telling you to grab a box and toss everything on those shelves, but you may want to consider pulling out the worst offenders and donating them to a shelter or local soup kitchen (it's not good mojo to throw out perfectly acceptable canned goods when so many people are starving).

Oh boy, did I hit the mother load when I viewed my own pantry from a pH standpoint for the first time. I knew that if these convenient foods were left on my shelves, I would find a way to sneak them into my diet.

Check your pantry or cupboards, and remove any of the following acid-provoking foods:

- Boxed or prepackaged meals
- Canned foods in creams or heavy syrups (legumes, vegetables, and fruits in no-sugar-added juice or water can stay)
- Crackers, bread, wheat pasta
- Chips, baked goods, peanut butter (or cheese) crackers, pretzels, (and any other snack-type food that does not grow on a tree
- Processed cereals
- White or brown rice

If a food item is processed or preserved in any way, more than likely it's an acid-forming food. Just think, when was the last time you saw cheese doodles growing on a tree? Have you ever picked plastic-wrapped peanut butter crackers off a bush? The majority of processed foods are acid-forming. When in doubt, eat foods in the form they were when picked from the tree, bush, or plant.

Clean out your pantry to provide more room for healthy, natural foods (and avoid reaching for comfortable old favorites).

Looking in your fridge

The biggest pH offenders in your icebox may be sitting on your condiment shelves.

Storing produce for long life

The next time you toss those spotted apples or gooey oranges in the trash consider how much money you are throwing away weekly in rotten produce.

- ✔ Bananas gone bad — $2.00
- ✔ Rotten apples — $4.00
- ✔ Bag of slimy spinach — $3.00
- ✔ Soft, brown oranges — $6.00

That's $15.00 in produce that needs to hit the trashcan. Fruits and vegetables are perishable, which means that natural enzymes and bacteria cause them to break down quickly and spoil. Instead of tossing all that used-to-be healthy food in the garbage, take a few minutes to protect your investment and keep your produce fresh.

If you bought your refrigerator after the dark ages you probably have crispers and humidity controls. The humidity control can be as simple as a slide on the drawer that you close for higher humidity or open for less humidity. Humidity equals moisture and moisture equals happy fruits and vegetables. Optimally, softer fruits and vegetables, such as greens, need a high humidity environment to stay fresh. Hard fruits and vegetables (think apples) survive well in a low humidity environment.

Keep your herbs fresh by storing their stems in a cup of water in the fridge, just like you would store fresh cut flowers. You can also dampen a paper towel and wrap it around stems of parsley, chives, or oregano to make the herbs last longer.

If you want to get ahead of the freshness game, buy from your local farm stand. Produce you buy at the grocery store has already traveled from the farm to the distribution center and from the distribution center to the store. You add days to produce's fridge life by cutting out the middleman.

Almost every condiment is a processed, convenient version of something you can make naturally. Think about ketchup — processed tomatoes with pounds of sugar. Or how about mayonnaise? Pulverized egg yolks and oil dripping with artery-clogging fats — I'd pass even if I wasn't watching my pH.

These acid-formers are commonly hiding in a refrigerator near you:

- ✔ Barbeque sauces or sautés
- ✔ Carbonated sodas
- ✔ Cheese, cream cheese, margarine, butter
- ✔ Jams, jellies, and syrup
- ✔ Ketchup
- ✔ Mayonnaise
- ✔ Salad dressings

If your hand starts shaking as you try to toss the mayo, don't worry, I have an excellent alkalinizing "mayo" recipe in Chapter 14.

Meat drawers are another source of acid-forming foods in your fridge. They are usually packed with hot dogs, luncheon meats, and bacon, none of which is good for your pH — not to mention your health. Processed meats are known to cause digestive cancers — fact, not fiction. Why play roulette with your digestive tract? These processed and cured meat concoctions shouldn't ever make it past your lips. I'm going to save the world . . . one strip of bacon at a time.

Diving into the freezer

If you have a "meat and potatoes" family, you may be assailed with racks of beef, lamb, and other frozen meat when you open the freezer door. This assortment can add up to hundreds of dollars, depending on the size of your freezer and how well it's stocked.

Except for skinless poultry and some seafood, such as salmon, the remaining meats in your fridge are most likely acid-forming and should be avoided on an acid alkaline diet.

Better than tossing all those animal products in the garbage, try to plan your acid alkaline diet start date around the time when the freezer will be vacated of all that acid-forming red meat. If you don't want to wait it out, consider throwing a big backyard party, grill the red meats, and feed them to the masses. Ta-da! — your freezer is now empty and ready to be stocked with less acid-forming foods (and I probably saved you points on your next cholesterol check).

Beware of the frozen meals as well; even the "healthy" freezer meals may be bursting with cheeses, fats, and acid-forming preservatives. When in doubt, donate them to your workplace freezer if you have one — some starving coworker is sure to nuke up your discarded freezer meals.

Shopping for the Right Stuff

Barring impending natural disasters, it's not hard to get your kitchen stocked with alkalinizing food choices — but it may be costly if you try to do it all at once. For starters, take a look at the list provided in Table 9-1, which provides a complete grocery list for every recipe in this book. You probably have a number of the ingredients already on hand!

Getting your staples

When I say staples, I'm not talking about the little metal clips used to bind paper — I'm speaking of the things you should always have on hand in your kitchen. Without these basic alkalinizing ingredients, it's very easy to fall back on old acidifying habits (exchanging refined white flour in a recipe that calls for spelt). Consider stocking up on:

- Basmati or wild rice
- Cold pressed olive oil
- Lentils
- Soy or almond milk
- Soy yogurt
- Spelt pastas
- Spelt, millet, or almond flour
- Sprouted grain bread or tortillas

Paired with the right fruits and vegetables, you can use these staples to make meals in place of the acidifying milk, flour, pasta, and bread that you may be using now.

Table 9-1 provides a helpful shopping list of acid-reducing foods.

Table 9-1	Acid Alkaline Grocery List			
Spices & Herbs	*Vegetables*	*Fruits & Juices*	*Proteins*	*Cooking Aids*
Allspice, Nutmeg	Cabbage	Bananas	Chicken breast	Alcohol-free vanilla extract
Basil	Carrots	Coconuts	Eggs	Apple cider vinegar
Bay leaves	Cauliflower	Fresh salsa	Egg substitute	Baking powder
Cayenne	Celery	Frozen or fresh strawberries	Lentils	Baking soda
Chili powder	Cooked pumpkin	Lemons	Pecans	Barley, Psyllium powder
Cilantro	Cucumbers	Lime juice	Pine nuts	Basmati or wild rice

Spices & Herbs	Vegetables	Fruits & Juices	Proteins	Cooking Aids
Cinnamon	Eggplant	Melons	Raw almonds	Butter (to make clarified butter)
Crushed red pepper flakes	Garlic	Oranges	Salmon	Clover honey
Cumin	Jalapenos	Pineapples	Shrimp	Cold-pressed olive oil
Dill weed	Kale, spinach, endive, butter lettuce	Tangerines	Soy or almond milk	Popcorn kernels
Dried chives	Mushrooms	Tomato juice	Soy powder	Quinoa
Garlic powder	Red/green bell peppers	Tomatoes	Soy yogurt	Rolled oats
Ginger	Scallions		Tofu (silken and firm)	Soy sauce
Oregano	Snow peas		Whey protein powder	Spelt pastas
Paprika	Sweet potatoes			Spelt, millet, or almond flour
Parsley	Yellow/red/white onions			Spicy V8
Pepper	Zucchini			Sprouted grain bread/tortillas
Peppercorns				Stevia
Rosemary				Tofutti Better Than Cream Cheese
Sea salt				Tomato sauce/paste
Thyme				Yeast-free vegetable broth

Filling up your fridge and freezer

After you clean out all the acidifying condiments and hairy oranges, it's time to restock your refrigerator with healthy, alkalinizing choices. More so than your cupboards, your fridge is the mainstay of a healthy acid alkaline diet. Fill your crispers and shelves with:

- Fresh produce (fruits, vegetables, herbs)
- Egg whites or perishable egg replacements
- Grains like quinoa and spelt pasta (if you live in the south, they need refrigeration)
- Dairy replacement products (almond milk, soy yogurt)

Replenish your frozen good selections with healthy, less acid-forming foods. Consider stocking it with choices such as:

- Flash frozen fruits and vegetables
- Salmon and skinless chicken breasts
- Soy yogurt (as an ice cream substitute)
- Fresh produce that you won't be using anytime soon

 If you buy produce in bulk, consider freezing half immediately after you get home. Unless you have a huge family, you're probably not going to eat an eight-pound bag of baby carrots in one sitting. Root vegetables and berries freeze well and taste the same upon defrosting, but lettuce and other leafy greens not so much. Keep sliced fruits and vegetables in airtight containers in the refrigerator. Many stores sell airtight plastic containers made specifically to keep produce fresh — a worthy investment in my mind.

Getting Past the Lame Excuses

Okay, so that heading sounds harsh, right? It's true. Most of us are extremely creative human beings who can come up with a lame excuse on the spot to rationalize our bad decisions. Some of my favorites include:

- I don't have time to cook.
- It's too expensive. (*It* being a healthy diet.)
- My family won't eat "rabbit food."
- My son only eats macaroni and cheese.
- Diets never work for me.

Choosing quality sea salt

You may have noticed that all of the recipes in this book call for sea salt. Completely different than plain old table salt, sea salt contains trace elements and minerals indigenous to the water from where it came. I've found salts from Hawaii, France, and Italy — all with varying colors, textures, and tastes (but you have to go to a gourmet store to find this kind of variety).

Using evaporation methods, sea salt is harvested from seawater, whereas table salt is mined from salt mines, chemically treated, and refined until only sodium chloride (salt) remains. Unlike table salt, some sea salts may contain trace amounts of healthy minerals including:

✔ Potassium

✔ Calcium

✔ Magnesium

✔ Bicarbonate

✔ Iron

✔ Manganese

✔ Zinc

Yes, it's more expensive than regular table salt, but the cost varies depending on your preference. The more exotic the sea salt (red, black, pink, smoked) the more it costs. You also pay more for the finely shaved "finishing" salts and kosher salts.

Regardless of what flavor or texture you desire, remember that it's still salt. You don't need more than 2,300 milligrams of the stuff per day (less than 1,500 milligrams if you have high blood pressure, kidney disease, or are black). Although that sounds like a lot, it only adds up to about a teaspoon daily depending on the coarseness of your sea salt.

Even if you're like me and always in a rush, eating healthy, alkalinizing foods can still be a part of your reality. Planning and time management are going to be your two new best friends from here on out. No more winging it and scarfing down fast food between work and social engagements. And no more lame excuses like, "It was the fast food or no food; I didn't have a choice." The next sections offer help in planning and managing meals for all types.

Whether you're a working adult, college student, or a really busy parent, if you eat anywhere other than in your home, consider investing in

✔ A thermal lunchbox or bag

✔ Re-usable ice blocks

✔ Airtight glass or plastic food containers

With these three tools, there's really no reason that healthy foods cannot become convenience foods. Just remember to use thermoses and ice blocks to keep your cold foods chilled and your hot foods warm — foodborne illnesses are not fun and they're often the product of improperly storing foods.

Feeling green around the gills? It could be what you ate

Food-borne illness, also called *food poisoning,* is a seriously under-diagnosed condition. Many people think they have a stomach bug and don't realize they've been afflicted with one of the dozens of germs that cause foodborne illness. Nausea, vomiting, and diarrhea can last up to a week or more after eating contaminated foods. Most normal, healthy adults can combat the bacteria naturally, however infants and young children, pregnant women, and the sick or elderly may need hospitalization and antibiotics to get rid of the bacteria causing the illness.

Contrary to popular belief, food poisoning is not caused only by eating raw meat, oysters, or dairy products. Foodborne illness can live on many different foods and surfaces including your hands and your countertops. Aside from raw animal products (eggs, meat), these diarrhea-cultivating germs can thrive on:

✔ Leafy greens

✔ Grains

✔ Fruits

✔ Nuts (including nut products like peanut butter)

Some of the most common pathogens causing this gastrointestinal distress include:

✔ Escheria coli (E. coli)

✔ Salmonella

✔ Campylobacter

✔ Shigella

✔ Clostridium

✔ Toxoplasma

✔ Listeria

✔ Staphylococcus

✔ Norovirus

The best way to avoid foodborne illness is to stop cross-contamination within your kitchen. Always wash your hands, counter tops, and kitchen utensils thoroughly. Keep raw products (poultry, fish, eggs) away from ready-to-eat products, such as sliced vegetables. Also, be sure to put leftovers away immediately. These germs thrive and multiply in room temperature foods. If you find cooked foods sitting on the counter one to two hours after dinner, don't take a chance with your gut — toss them out!

Planning for convenience

Pick a day of the week, and make it your meal planning and cooking day. (My mother-in-law taught me this priceless tip.) When her children were young, she would prepare meals for the entire week and freeze them. After all, it's just as easy to have three pots boiling on the stove as it is to have just one!

I have a four-person family. The average person eats at least three meals a day, which adds up to 84 meals per week. No way I'm preparing 84 meals in advance — not to mention where in the world would I store them? I only cook our dinners in advance — seven large meals is a lot more manageable than 84 small ones.

Many of the dinner recipes mentioned in Chapter 15 freeze well. I like to make the Stuffed Green Peppers ahead of time and freeze them individually. That way, I can eat one for lunch or I can thaw them all for a quick and tasty family dinner.

Chapter 15 contains a recipe for alkaline forming pizza dough. Make it ahead of time and freeze the raw dough. Take the dough out of the freezer in the morning and put it in the refrigerator to thaw. Now you have the base for a quick dinner when you get home.

Take your routine into account while meal planning for the week. We enjoy smoothies or granola for breakfast, and I pack leftovers for school and work lunches.

Managing your time

Make time to eat a healthy diet through time management. Sure, it would be a lot faster to nuke hot dogs as opposed to cooking a nice, fresh meal in the 15 minutes between school and ball games, but you can easily prepare ahead of time for the after-school rush.

Only you know the idiosyncrasies of your family's routines and schedules. I usually have a pretty good idea of what my next week is going to look like and you probably do too. So, slice, dice, and sauté up meals and snacks ahead of time if next week is booked with engagements.

Calculating Costs

I want to debunk my favorite healthy diet argument: I can't eat healthy because it's too expensive! Seeing the rising cost of fresh produce and taking into account some of the specialty products you may use on the acid alkaline diet (soy milk, tofu, spelt pastas), an alkalinizing diet is still economically better for your wallet than eating processed foods and going to restaurants.

The trick is in knowing how to buy, store, and use your foods wisely. Stroll the aisles of the grocery store, and you may be surprised to find that processed foods are actually more expensive than the raw or natural foods you need to be eating. Don't believe me? Bag of cheese doodles: $3.75. Bag of apples: $2.50. Other ways to manage costs include:

✔ **Eat out less frequently.** Although you can eat out on the acid alkaline diet, you probably shouldn't make it a habit. Eating out is more expensive than cooking your own meals at home (and you may not have the great leftovers for lunch tomorrow).

- ✔ **Decrease food waste.** Just because you can buy a ten-pound bag of onions with a coupon this week, are you really going to eat all ten pounds before they spoil? Unless you're expecting a hurricane, stick to buying what you need for the week (excluding toilet paper — apparently you can never have too much of that).

- ✔ **Be a store connoisseur.** Unless you own stock in the company, you should have no loyalty to any one particular store. Shop where prices are the cheapest and the produce is the freshest because, after all, the majority of your acid alkaline purchases are made in the produce department.

- ✔ **Watch your receipts.** Cashiers are people, and they make mistakes. If your bill seems a little high, don't hesitate to question it. Also, pay attention to the price of goods as you buy them. If the price of bananas is climbing this month, it may be time to switch to another fruit (it helps add variety to your diet, as well).

Shopping one week at a time

You can save money by planning your weekly shopping, then sticking to the plan. Cut coupons, compare prices by stores, read circulars, and don't shop when the mood hits you. I've found that I spend almost twice as much on groceries in one month if I go to the store more often than once per week.

I know this sounds cliché, but don't shop when you're hungry. Convenient food items will call to you and your willpower may waver. There's a reason that they call those items in the checkout line *impulse buys* — you're more likely to buy one of those chocolate bars or cans of chilled soda while you're standing there waiting in line.

Stick to your shopping list. If the items you think you so desperately want aren't on it, don't buy them.

Keep a list on the fridge and use it. As you cook and deplete your food supply, add the items to your list immediately. (I actually keep my running list on my cellphone so I am never away from home without it.)

Getting the most out of leftovers

You may be making a face right now at the word *leftovers*. But leftovers are an excellent way to keep more of your hard-earned cash by finishing the foods you already prepared instead of going out to buy more.

When they are safely stored in the refrigerator at or under 40 degrees Fahrenheit, leftovers are usually safe to consume up to four days following the meal. Get a strip of masking tape and a permanent marker; you can use the tape to label leftovers with the date you put them in the fridge. Don't judge a food's safety by smell or taste alone — the germs that cause food-borne illness don't initially alter the food's outward appearance but they will get you sick.

If you live alone or have a small family, you can split a meal the minute it comes out of the oven. I've done it with a huge tray of vegetarian lasagna that tasted even better when I reheated it! If you know you won't eat the entire meal, go ahead and store half of it in the freezer the minute it's cool enough.

Getting the Family on Board

You've got a plan to eat right, exercise, and dump the acids out of your body to regain your health and well-being. What about the rest of your family? Unless you live alone, you may want to bring them on board with the plan, too.

Talk to your doctor if you have concerns about the nutrition requirements of small children, sick family members, or the elderly.

Don't park it in front of the boob tube

I read a devastating statistic the other day, scarier than any horror flick I've seen lately. A survey of American children showed infants watch about two hours of TV per day on average. Holy cow! Kids have plenty of time to develop their media skills and will be texting and playing on the Internet soon enough. Getting too much daily TV time can put children at risk for:

- Decreased social skills (difficulty making friends)

- Slower brain development (less interaction with the world around them)

- Decreased physical development (not running, skipping, and playing outside)

- Poor academics (not doing homework in favor of TV)

- Obesity and overweight (sedentary lifestyle)

- Desensitization to violent acts (as seen on TV)

Similarly, adults who watch a few hours of television daily increase all of the risks associated with a sedentary lifestyle including obesity. Hit the Off button on that remote and engage your children in an epic water balloon fight, bike ride through the neighborhood, or go on a nature hike. Most likely, your children will find those events far more fascinating than the latest episode of *Pookie the Deranged Space Monkey*, and they get to spend time with their favorite person: you.

Converting kids to healthy foods

As you progress in your acid alkaline diet and lifestyle, your children probably won't be thrilled to see that the pantry is devoid of processed snack foods. If you can maintain your willpower to avoid them, it's not a bad idea to slowly wean children off of their beloved crunchy-o's or sugary puffs instead of making them quit cold turkey. Some methods that succeed — at least sometimes — include:

- **Teach with subterfuge:** Consider talking to your children about the food choices while you cook or chop fruits and veggies. Discuss things like how red the tomatoes are or how soft the apricots feel. Most kids don't appreciate lectures on the vitamin and nutritional content of healthy foods, but they can and do appreciate tastes, textures, and appearance.

- **Patience, patience, patience:** You can begin to offer healthy alternatives to their usual snacks and slowly introduce them to new veggies on their dinner plate. Substitute a pretty plate of chopped carrots with a new dip for greasy chips or make a smiley face out of a sprouted grain tortilla and give it a cream cheese replacement mustache. I had to put spinach on my younger son's plate at least five times before he finally accepted it as a normal part of his dinner (and ate it!).

- **Take charge:** I know how easy it is to cave in the pleading face of a four-year-old, but don't do it! As a parent I take my role very seriously. Until they can drive (and maybe even after), you are the gatekeeper of your children's nutrition. If you don't buy it, they can't eat it.

Leading the pack

Even if your partner or children are not on board with your acid alkaline diet plan, you can lead by example. If your partner witnesses your increased vitality, energy, and weight loss, he or she is sure to start showing some interest.

If that doesn't work, you can try talking to your reluctant spouse. He or she may not fully understand your reasoning behind the diet. Perhaps after you explain that you love your spouse, and that optimally you want to be healthy and grow old together, he or she may be more receptive to trying something new.

Worst-case scenario, if your family is not interested in joining the acid alkaline diet train, you don't have to force it on them. Even if they want to continue eating red meat or dairy products, they can benefit from additional helpings of veggies and fresh fruit from your stash.

Chapter 10

Talking to Your Doctor

Your doctor is a vital part of your healthcare team. A partner in your wellness, he or she is there to help you make better decisions to maintain or repair damaged health and to lead you back to wellbeing in times of illness. I'm sure that's not the definition you'll see for a doctor when you check a dictionary, but as a nurse for over 15 years, it works for me.

Consult your doctor prior to making any dietary or lifestyle changes. The whole, "better to ask forgiveness rather than permission" adage only works with your spouse and close friends. If you suffer a chronic illness or medical problem, I wrote this chapter especially for you. Although the majority of recommendations in this book are intended for healthy, average adults, I realize that a number of people seeking the benefits of the acid alkaline diet may not fit in this category.

Your body is a synergistic machine. Everything you put in your mouth, including medications and food, has an effect on you. This chapter shows you how foods, medications, and even over-the-counter pills can effect your acid-base balance.

Setting Up a Visit with Your Doctor

Before you get a chance to talk to your doctor about altering your diet, you need to arrange an appointment. Depending on your insurance coverage, you can go about this a few different ways: If you're on a Health Maintenance Organization (HMO) insurance plan, you have a primary physician who manages all your care, and any questions about diet or medications need to be addressed with your primary physician; if you have a Preferred Provider

Organization (PPO) plan, you have the option of choosing a doctor to discuss your nutritional needs.

I use the term *chronic medical condition* quite frequently throughout this chapter. The term is relevant to anyone receiving ongoing medical treatment. Your chronic medical condition may include taking a pill every day for high blood pressure or impending back surgery for a herniated disc (and so many things in between those two extremes).

I'm not sitting there beside you — I don't know if you have a medical condition. All I can do is strongly encourage you to talk to your doctor before starting a dietary change if you do.

Gaining your doctor's approval

With a chronic medical condition, approval to modify your diet should occur in a face-to-face meeting with your doctor. I know, I know — that's inconvenient. But your doctor needs to physically see and assess you. He or she may want to order blood tests to check your:

- ✔ Electrolytes
- ✔ Kidney function
- ✔ Pancreas (blood sugar regulation)
- ✔ Liver
- ✔ Cholesterol and triglycerides (fats in the blood)

Debunking myths

Although I don't have statistics, I'm reasonably sure that a number of physicians aren't fully familiar with the acid alkaline diet and lifestyle. Here are some of the most common misconceptions I hear when people ask me (or tell me their thoughts) about the acid alkaline diet:

- ✔ **It's used to treat acid reflux (heartburn).** Well, yes and no. Although the same foods and beverages that can elicit a nasty bout of heartburn *are* discouraged on the acid alkaline diet, it's not the same as a GERD (gastroesophageal reflux disease) diet. GERD diets reduce acid-stimulating foods

(in your stomach, not your body) such as citrus, tomatoes, chocolate, mint, and caffeine.

- ✔ **It's a fad.** Eating right and exercising is not a fad. If I encouraged you to inject yourself, eat only grapefruit, or knock out entire food groups — well now that would be a fad diet.

- ✔ **I can never eat an "acidic" food again.** Again, not true. The idea is to decrease the amounts of acid-forming foods you ingest, not eliminate them completely.

Your doctor may also document your blood pressure, heart rate, height, and weight. He or she can review your medications and current condition and discuss how changing your diet may affect you.

The reason you want this adventure documented? If you have a pre-existing medical condition, such as obesity, your health and life insurance premiums may drop if your weight loss and healthy habits are documented. Check with your providers to be sure — it only takes a phone call to find out and possibly save you money.

Starting a discussion

Arrive at your doctor's office prepared. Have a checklist of questions or concerns at the ready, and use your brief time with the physician wisely. You should also bring (to every visit) a list of your medications including any over-the-counter pills or nutritional supplements that you take. Consider asking your doctor:

- Is an acid alkaline diet right for me? Why or why not?
- Could this diet possibly aggravate my [insert medical condition here]?
- (If you're overweight) How much weight do I need to lose to be at a safe, healthy weight for my body shape?
- Can you provide an exercise regiment to get me started?
- Do you recommend I see a nutritionist or registered dietician?
- How often should I follow up with you?

Abiding by your doctor's wishes

Although it's highly unlikely that your doctor says, "No, Mrs. Smith. You shouldn't start the acid alkaline diet and eat more fruits, vegetables, and healthy proteins," it's possible.

You don't want to argue with your physician, but you may feel the need to educate him or her. With the plethora of trendy diets available, it's always possible that your doctor doesn't know much about the acid alkaline diet (or just calls it eating healthy and never realized it had a name).

I'll throw in a caveat and say that there may be a perfectly good reason your doctor doesn't want you changing your diet at this time. For instance, if you're scheduled for major surgery or have chronic kidney problems, your doctor may have you on a very special diet calculated to meet your needs. In these cases, you can ask your doctor how to incorporate more alkalinizing food choices while still adhering to your prescribed diet.

Examining Chronic Conditions

Since chronic conditions range from toenail fungus to chronic obstructive pulmonary disease (COPD), I'm only going to hit on the conditions most impacted when it comes to altering your diet.

If you have diabetes, heart disease, or kidney disease, you're probably already on a special diet and may have consulted with a registered dietician or nutritionist. Speak to that medical professional prior to proceeding.

Digging into diabetes

In general, diabetes is a disorder of your body's sugar metabolism. Depending on what type of diabetes you have, you may be unable to produce *insulin,* a hormone that helps regulate the sugar in your blood, on your own, or your body may be unable to properly use the insulin you have.

Your doctor's dietary recommendations vary depending on which type of diabetes you have:

✔ Gestational (during pregnancy)

✔ Type 1 (previously called *juvenile* or *insulin-dependent diabetes*)

✔ Type 2 (used to be referred to as *adult onset diabetes,* although some obese children are impacted by type 2 diabetes now as well)

Carbohydrates, the sugars that make up starches, sweets, and fiber, impact your blood sugar — some more than others. Blood sugar spikes that look like a roller coaster (high, low, high, low) are unsafe for your health. Adhering to a diet with diabetes is easier than it used to be because there's greater understanding of which carbs impact people the most and how to avoid blood-sugar spikes.

The old-fashioned caloric limitations have been lifted off of most diabetics (some people with advanced type 1 diabetes may still have certain restrictions due to the nature of their disease) and a pattern of healthy eating put in its place.

The acid alkaline diet pairs nicely with most diabetic nutritional instructions. People with diabetes are encouraged to limit intake of

✔ Fatty and processed meats

✔ Fatty foods

✔ Sweets and sodas

Hmm. Isn't that interesting — a person eating the acid alkaline diet is discouraged to eat those foods as well! Diabetics are encouraged to eat more

- ✔ Lean meats, such as chicken and fish
- ✔ Natural fibers, such as those found in fruits and vegetables, nuts and seeds

Your doctor or dietician uses your blood sugar as a guide to your dietary recommendations. If you blood sugar remains high or uncontrolled, he or she may tell you to reduce the amount of carbohydrates you consume daily. Your doctor or nurse can work closely with you and help you make healthy exchanges in the acid alkaline diet. For instance, she may discourage eating as much fruit (fruit has natural sugars that impact blood sugar) and encourage upping your lean proteins or fiber (vegetables, nuts, seeds) intake. Working with your doctor or nutritionist, you can enjoy a healthy, alkalinizing lifestyle.

Leaving gluten alone if you have celiac disease

You can absolutely adhere to an acid alkaline diet with celiac disease. This disease of the small intestine interferes with your body's ability to digest *gluten,* a protein found in barley, wheat, oats, rye, and products made with those grains. I've even found gluten in lip balm — so avoiding it's a little more challenging that the non-celiac sufferer might think.

Many of the recipes I provide for an acid alkaline diet include gluten or gluten derivatives. A little creativity and you can make them gluten free in no time. Avoid or alter the recipes that include:

- ✔ Barley
- ✔ Bulgur
- ✔ Spelt (flour or pasta)

Instead of those celiac antagonists, consider using:

- ✔ Amaranth
- ✔ Millet or soy flour
- ✔ Quinoa

Celiac sufferers are encouraged to make fruits, vegetables, and lean proteins a healthy part of their diet. Good news — that's what the majority of the acid alkaline diet is composed of!

Make sure you always check labels and read ingredients if you are making any of my recipes. They're composed of fruits and vegetables for the most part, but I wouldn't want to accidentally mislead you and I cannot guarantee that there isn't some form of gluten called for in a recipe.

Fighting irritable bowel

The person who suffers irritable bowel disease (IBD, not to be confused with Irritable Bowel Syndrome, IBS) knows that a moment of sugary satisfaction is not worth the pain and suffering that follows it. Crohn's disease and ulcerative colitis are two diseases categorized as IBD, which may cause abdominal pain, bloating, diarrhea, and even blood or mucus in the stools.

For some IBD sufferers any or all of the following can stimulate an uncomfortable symptom flare-up:

- ✓ Alcohol
- ✓ Caffeine
- ✓ Dairy products
- ✓ Sugar

Of course this list is not all-inclusive — many other things can stimulate an IBD flare-up as well, but these are the most popular. When your symptoms are out of control, your doctor may place you on a special diet that gives your digestive tract time to rest. You may be put on a

- ✓ Low or reduced fiber diet
- ✓ Clear or full liquid diet

Although fiber can occasionally be your enemy, talk to your doctor about how to incorporate healthy, alkalinizing foods into your dietary regiment without suffering for it.

Working with food allergies

Food sensitivities, also known as food allergies, are the result of an overactive immune system. The body of a person with a food allergy reacts to certain foods no differently than it does to a germ — it goes on full red alert and over-reacts to get rid of the offending food.

There is no cure for food allergies. If anything, your sensitivity to the food may increase, and the next time you eat the offending food your reaction may be worse. You may start with itchy eyes or a dripping nose, but the next time you may get hives covering your body. Worst case scenario, if you eat a food you are truly allergic to, your throat and vocal cords can swell up — an emergency situation that requires immediate medical care.

Although you can technically be allergic to anything, common culprits for food allergies include

- ✔ Fish and shellfish
- ✔ Milk and eggs
- ✔ Nuts
- ✔ Wheat and soybeans

If you have a known allergy to any of these foods (or any others, for that matter), don't tempt fate by eating them. It's best to schedule a visit with an *immunologist* or *allergist,* the doctors that specialize in food allergies.

You can still enjoy a healthy, alkalinizing diet with food allergies if you're mindful of the food (or food group) that you must avoid.

Don't try to guess or take a chance eating a specific food again if you suspect you have a food allergy. Even seemingly innocuous symptoms can become severe in a matter of minutes.

Paying attention to heart disease

There are a couple different variations of diets for people suffering heart disease such as the DASH (Dietary Approaches to Stop Hypertension) diet, low-fat diet, and sodium (salt) restricted diets.

Your risk of heart disease is directly linked to your diet (among other factors like your genes, activity level, and lifestyle). The easiest way to keep your heart happy is by enjoying a nutritious, low-fat diet rich with healthy ingredients.

Pretty much everything you need to avoid or limit on the acid alkaline diet should be avoided or limited on a heart-healthy diet as well.

Talk with your doctor to incorporate the acid alkaline diet into your heart-healthy diet. He or she may encourage:

- ✔ Five daily servings of fruits and vegetables
- ✔ Decreased bad fats on the diet (using less clarified butter)
- ✔ Increased grains (alkalinizing ones like wild rice, quinoa)

Avoid the unhealthy fats like cholesterol and trans and saturated fats. These are the fats loaded into red meat and basic cooking oils — so you're already a step ahead when you drop those from your diet. Plus, turning to lean proteins like fish offers your heart those exciting heart-healthy fats called omega-3s.

Tackling obesity

Obesity is diagnosed when you are grossly overweight. It's not a condition to be taken lightly, as it's associated with many chronic diseases including heart problems, diabetes type 2, and joint degeneration. Barring any genetic disorders causing it, your diet and nutrition are important parts of treating obesity.

I read a study that said people who are obese schedule more annual doctor's appointments than smokers, but what does that mean for the people who are obese and smoke? That's something to think about.

Unless you're cheating, it's probably going to be difficult to stay overweight on a largely plant-based diet. Many of the acid-forming foods are also the culprits to unintentional weight gain. Table 10-1 shows how many calories can be dropped daily just by cutting out some of these acidifying offenders.

Table 10-1	Cutting Acids and Calories
Acid-forming Food	*Calories*
12-ounce can of non-diet cola	136
Hamburger with condiments	294
One serving of fries (vary by brand)	203

The calorie counts are approximate, based on data from the United States Agricultural Department's Nutrition Data Laboratory.

Dropping a pound a week

So you lost 13 pounds in three weeks? That's super, but there's a projected downside: Chances are, you'll gain that weight (and more) back again unless you lost it through *gastric bypass* (a surgery to lose weight). You're encouraged to lose one to two pounds a week maximum to make the change stick. That's an eight-pound weight loss per month, tops. If that doesn't sound like much then I'd say you've never lost eight pounds.

Celebrate each pound lost. There's a positive correlation between the amount of weight you lose and the amount of stress that comes off your joints. If you drop even one pound, you also drop the pressure you place on your knees and lower back. This reduces your risk of arthritis, herniated discs, and general wear and tear on your body.

Losing a pound a week may occur naturally once you embark on a healthy, sugar-free diet. Experts say that one pound is equal to 3,500 calories (that's 500 calories a day). If you used to drink sugary soft drinks or have bagels for breakfast, cutting those items out of your diet alone will probably drop your daily intake by 500 calories.

The other thing to think about while you're looking at Table 10-1 — not too many people have just a 12-ounce soda, a plain ketchup and mayo burger, or a normal serving of French fries. The meal example I used totaled 633 calories with proper serving sizes, and if you up the size of that meal, you up the calories.

Talk to your doctor if you've had gastric surgery for obesity. The surgeon is responsible for watching your diet and nutrient intake, monitoring how well you tolerate the system, and progressing the diet for you.

Reading Medication Labels

When was the last time you sat and read the multi-page pamphlet that comes with your medications? These pamphlets provide a virtual jackpot of information about the medication and shouldn't hit the trash the second you get home. Drug information sheets can tell you:

- ✔ How to take the medication
- ✔ What it's used for
- ✔ What to do if you miss a dose
- ✔ How to store it
- ✔ What medications it may interact with
- ✔ What foods or beverages can hamper its efficacy

Caffeine is a drug

Believe it — caffeine is a drug. It's a natural stimulant found in coffee beans, tea leaves, and even cocoa. It's a stimulant drug, meaning it excites the central nervous system. This is why that cup of java in the morning wakes you up or that afternoon soda gives you an energy burst.

However, you can have too much of a good thing. Caffeine is hidden in many energy drinks, supplements, and even medications (think over-the-counter headache medicine). If you don't keep tabs on your daily dosage you could end up with:

✔ Jitters

✔ Anxiety or feeling nervous

✔ Nauseous

✔ Increased blood pressure and heart rate

How much can you tolerate? Although experts recommend keeping your caffeine intake less than 400 milligrams per day (that's about four small cups of coffee brewed at home), your caffeine tolerance depends on your size, metabolism, activity, and how much of the stuff you take in. Like any stimulant drug, you can actually develop a tolerance to caffeine. This means that you may need more and more of it to feel the uplifting effects on your energy.

Food-drug interactions

Some medications don't play well with certain foods or beverages. If you take them together, you run the risk of either rendering the drug ineffective or, worse yet, magnifying the drug's effect so it becomes far more potent than it should be. The technical name for this is a drug's *bioavailability* — some chemicals in food and drink impact the amount of drug that's available for absorption by your body.

The following is by no means an all-inclusive list, but some of the most common drug and food interactions stem from taking certain prescription medications along with:

✔ Alcohol

✔ Caffeine

✔ Cranberry juice

✔ Avocado

✔ Grapefruit or grapefruit juice

✔ Dark green leafed vegetable (spinach, kale)

Cranberry juice and avocados have the potential to increase the effects of *warfarin,* a prescription blood thinner. Grapefruits and grapefruit juice (and some citrus for that matter) have the potential to interact with medications for your heart, depression, anxiety, immune system suppression, seizures, and even cholesterol-lowering drugs (*statins*). My point is, although they are healthy, natural foods, they may not be the best alkalinizing choice for you. Only you and your doctor can decide which foods work best with your pre-scribed medications.

If you've already tossed the drug information pamphlet and now have a question about a food-drug interaction for your medications, contact the prescribing doctor or the pharmacist.

Keeping a medication list

Keep a list of the medications you take daily, especially if you visit multiple doctors. There's always a chance that your physicians don't talk to one another, and therefore have no knowledge of what the other provider ordered. When I say medications, I mean every pill, dietary, or herbal supplement that passes your lips.

Keep a list of everything you take with you so that you can show it to anyone who prescribes or otherwise recommends medications or supplements. Include the following information on your list:

- ✔ The name of the medication or supplement
- ✔ What it treats or why you take it
- ✔ The dosage amount and how often you take it
- ✔ The delivery method — whether by mouth, injection, inhalation
- ✔ The name of the prescribing medical professional

Chapter 11

Figuring Out What You Can Eat

All right you list lovers, I wrote this chapter just for you. It's stuffed full of charts depicting specific foods and their potential to be acid or alkaline-forming foods after you eat them. Put away your litmus paper — a food's acidity or alkalinity prior to digestion has no impact on how it affects your body and pH.

Back in Chapter 4, I said that we are all different creatures — what impacts my pH may not impact yours. However, certain foods are known to increase acidity in most people, whereas others can help alkalinize your body. I'm not a biochemist, so these lists are formed from my knowledge base of acid and alkaline-forming foods as well as personal experience. The bottom line: These lists are fluid and should be used as a basic guideline, not holy doctrine.

Even if you're the kind of person who cannot stand foods touching on your plate, they all merge after you swallow. Foods have a synergistic effect, meaning they sometimes work together in your body to create a combined effect. Think about calcium and vitamin D; you must have one to reap the benefits of the other.

 Understanding and living a pH-driven diet doesn't have to become a chemistry experiment in your kitchen. You can eat anything you want, you just have to realize that some acid-forming foods are so detrimental to your pH that they should be relegated to special occasions.

Loving the Alkalinizing Foods

I want to start off this chapter with lists of the healthy, alkalinizing foods you can eat. The foods in these sections are the ones you want to fill your plate with. Things aren't all joyful, however, I follow up the good news with comparable lists of foods to eat sparingly, if at all, in the upcoming "Avoiding Acid-Forming Foods" section.

Acid alkaline dieting is not an exact science — select the majority of your foods out of the following lists and you're sure to at least improve your pH — and probably your health and well-being as well.

Selecting the best fruit

Some fruits are good for your pH, and some fruits are really good for your pH. When you're slicing and dicing for a fruit tray (because I know that's what you're having for dessert tonight) consider picking some of the very alkaline-forming fruits in this list:

- ✔ **Least alkalinizing:** Apple, banana, blueberries, orange, strawberry, tomato

- ✔ **Moderately alkalinizing:** Apricot, grapefruit, honeydew, peach, pear, tropical fruits such as kiwi, mango, papaya, and star fruit

- ✔ **Very alkalinizing:** Avocado, cantaloupe, lemon, lime, pineapple, tangerines, watermelon

Any of these fruits is a better choice than the more acid-forming fruits listed in the upcoming "Minimizing acid-forming fruits" section, so choose fruits from this list.

Stocking up on the right veggies

Honestly, you can't really go wrong with fresh vegetables on the acid alkaline diet. With so many varieties, colors, and textures to choose from, it's still a wonder to me that more plates aren't covered in what my friends lovingly call "rabbit food." I think our guinea pig had it right — she was an herbivore and ate her weight in fresh veggies daily (boy, was her coat shiny).

For an out-of-this-world alkaline pH, the majority of your daily intake should come from the "Very alkalinizing" category of this list:

- ✔ **Least alkalinizing:** Artichoke, celery, leek, lettuce (it's mostly water), okra, scallions

- ✔ **Moderately alkalinizing:** Asparagus, cauliflower, celery, parsley, spinach

- ✔ **Very alkalinizing:** Bell peppers, broccoli, cabbage, eggplant, endive, garlic, kale, lentils, mustard greens, onion, pumpkin, seaweed, sweet potato

Getting picky about proteins

If you've already perused the recipe chapters, you know that I'm a big fan of mixing up proteins. I like to keep things real — I love tofu, but I don't want to live off of the stuff.

The following list shows the top alkaline-forming proteins so that you can experiment with more than chicken and salmon.

- **Least alkalinizing:** Egg whites, egg replacements, whey protein powder

- **Moderately alkalinizing:** Almond milk, seeds such as flax seeds, pumpkin seeds, and sunflower seeds, soy yogurt, soy milk

- **Very alkalinizing:** Almonds and chestnuts; fermented soy as in tofu, tempeh, and miso; all sprouts; lentils

There's an exception to every rule. Although the majority of naturally grown plant foods are alkalinizing, most nuts are the exception. You may have noticed that the majority of beloved nuts didn't make this list — that's intentional. Nuts are always a better choice for your pH than say, a steak, but some popular favorites, such as peanuts, brazil nuts, and pistachios, are acid-forming.

Try to introduce new proteins a few at a time into your meal plans. The seeds and nuts work great as snacks, whereas protein powders, silken tofu, and egg whites spruce up omelets and soups.

The roof of my mouth is all itchy

Actually, oral allergy syndrome (OAS) can make any part of your mouth itchy including your tongue and lips, not just the roof of your mouth. OAS is not the same thing as a true food allergy — it's a sensitivity to the pollen that binds with fruit, nuts, or vegetables.

The response is usually limited to your mouth, and you probably won't have the same response if you eat the food again cooked. Cooking the food destroys the pollen, hence no itchies. However, OAS can potentially transform into a real food allergy, so it's a good idea to see your doctor if you suspect you have an intolerance to certain produce.

People who suffer hay fever or seasonal allergies usually know exactly what type of pollen is causing their misery. The three main offenders, birch, grass, and ragweed, have counterparts that you may be sensitive to as well:

- If you have a **grass allergy,** you may be sensitive to potatoes and tomatoes.

- If you have a **birch (tree) allergy,** you may be sensitive to almonds, apples, carrots, hazelnuts, pears, or plums.

- If you have a **ragweed allergy**, you may be sensitive to bananas, cucumbers, melons, or zucchinis.

Selecting grains, nuts, and oils

With so many different grain products facing you at the store, sticking to your acid alkaline diet may seem challenging at times.

Focus on the things that you want to eat to balance your pH, not the things that you should avoid. Instead of saying, "I wish I could have that tuna on whole wheat toast," think to yourself, "Tuna on a sprouted grain tortilla is going to be tasty!" Okay, so maybe I'm stretching your tolerance, but you'll get there.

The healthy, alkaline-forming grains, nuts, and oils that should fill your pantry include

- ✔ **Least alkalinizing:** Barley, millet, pine nuts, quinoa, rolled oats, spelt, triticale, wild rice
- ✔ **Moderately alkalinizing:** Chestnuts, cod liver oil, flax seeds, poppy seeds, pumpkin seeds
- ✔ **Very alkalinizing:** Almonds, avocado oil, cold-pressed olive oil, sprouted grains including sprouted bread and tortillas

Getting good "dairy"

Excluding *ghee,* which is clarified butter, use dairy products sparingly on a pH balanced diet. The majority of dairy products, although tasty, are acid-forming. Unless you have an exchange on hand, this can prove to be a problem when cooking since many recipes call for milk, eggs, cheese, or butter.

You can find plenty of dairy replacement products at the grocery store, which are usually hiding in the health food section by the tofu. Stock your fridge with these alkalinizing dairy substitutes:

- ✔ **Least alkalinizing:** Egg whites, egg replacement products, ghee (clarified butter), whey protein (isolated milk derivative)
- ✔ **Moderately alkalinizing:** Almond milk, soy cheese, soy milk, soy yogurt

Drumming up hidden alkaline-formers

When I started thinking about the miscellaneous items that are alkaline-forming, the first to spring to mind was breast milk. Ha! Good luck finding that one in the grocer's aisles. But just think about that — the first thing babies need and survive on (some exclusively) is breast milk.

When you're looking to add a little hidden pH booster to snacks and meals, the substances listed here should do the trick. Sometimes it's the simple things that turn an okay snack into an alkalinizing one!

> ✔ **Least alkalinizing:** Aloe vera, clover honey
>
> ✔ **Moderately alkalinizing:** Algae, ginger and herbal teas, stevia
>
> ✔ **Very alkalinizing:** Apple cider vinegar, baking soda, green tea, lemon water, mineral water, sea salt

Avoiding Acid-Forming Foods

Even foods that you think of as healthy may have some acidifying effects in your body. The trick is to memorize the biggest offenders and use them sparingly — if at all — in your kitchen.

The acid alkaline diet doesn't eliminate whole food groups from your diet. It's about making better choices for your overall pH. You can still eat acid-forming foods, but you have to pay attention to how many of them fill your plate at each sitting.

Minimizing acid-forming fruits

I'll admit, the concept I struggled the most with on an acid alkaline diet was that certain fruits are actually acid-forming, and therefore, not so good for your pH.

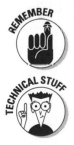

I'm not saying fruit is bad for you, but every fruit contains naturally occurring sugars, which form acid during digestion. There are shades of gray here — fruits are not equal in their sugar content.

A fruit's acid-forming potential is dependent on its caloric density, or how many calories are packed into each bite of the fruit. Watery fruits tend to have a lower caloric density and therefore a lower acid-forming potential, whereas dried and dense fruits have higher calorie content — and therefore more acid-forming potential. Grapes and raisins — same fruit, right? Not so. One cup of grapes has 104 calories, which is much lower than the 493 calories a cup of raisins has. Even the cute little snack packs of raisins have more calories than a cup of grapes! It's truly not the size that matters; it's the caloric density of the food.

Sprucing up your fruit life

Getting tired of the melons and bananas? Extend your cultural reach at the produce market (or dazzle your friends) with your fruit knowledge. Nature's bounty provides so much more than the typical staples we're used to seeing at the grocery store. The majority of tropical fruits are alkaline-forming, but citrus has the potential to be mildly acid-forming due to its high sugar content. When in doubt, try them sparingly, like in a dessert dish. Next time you need a fruit pick-me-up, consider trying

✔ **Blowfish fruit:** I can't help it; I call the Kiwano melon by its American name because it looks like a blowfish. This fruit has a burnt orange peel with spikes covering the surface. It has a cantaloupe-colored inside (and a mild melon taste) and is filled with edible gooey-green seeds.

✔ **Blood orange:** If you're a fan of the American TV show *Dexter,* you've seen these frightening fruits in the intro. Blood oranges are aptly named for their dark red pulp and juice, which appears almost bloody in comparison to the bright orange

outer skin. Don't let it scare you off, the fruit packs a vitamin C punch and tastes delicious.

✔ **Dragon fruit:** This flaming pink fruit is commonly used as a flavorful drink ingredient, but have you actually ever seen one? A more accurate name, pitaya, is indigenous to South and Central America. It has tiny black seeds similar to those in a kiwi fruit with a mild, sweet flavored flesh.

✔ **Prickly pear:** Or you could call it the Indian fig, cactus fruit, or even cactus pear — whatever name you give it, this delicious fruit tastes of cucumbers and mild watermelon with its sweet reddish flesh. Serve it cold, but don't eat the skin — it has tiny prickers!

✔ **Star fruit:** I have to admit I had the plastic version of these in a bowl for two years before I saw the real thing at the produce market. These waxy yellow and green fruits taste of pineapple and lemon and look like a five-pointed star when chopped horizontally (hence the name).

The following list identifies some of the other fruits that can negatively impact your pH:

✔ **Least acid forming:** Coconut, dates

✔ **Moderately acid forming:** Plums, cherries, prunes, and other dried fruits including raisins

✔ **Very acid forming:** Pomegranate, cranberries, blackberries, and processed fruits such as those in marmalades and jams

You may notice that I use some of these fruits in my recipes in Part IV — the trick is using them sparingly and almost always in their natural form.

Always try to eat the real, natural fruit, not the processed stuff, to protect your pH. Take coconut for example: Dried, shaved coconut is more acid-forming than the stuff you carve from the hairy fruit.

Declaring acid-forming veggies

I hate to say it, but certain veggies (some of my favorites) have the potential to form an acid ash during digestion. Similar to their fruit buddies, the most offending veggies are usually the ones you love because they have simple sugars and taste great without a lot of culinary imagination.

When picking your produce, your pH will be happier if you eat the vegetables in this list less often:

- **Least acid forming:** Kidney beans, string beans, navy beans, black-eyed peas, green peas

- **Moderately acid forming:** Carrots, green beans, lima beans, chick peas, snow peas, split peas

- **Very acid forming:** Corn, white potatoes

Tossing the acid-forming proteins

You need protein in your diet — that's non-negotiable. This little molecule is the starter for almost every cell in your body from your hair to your liver. Protein is used to repair and regenerate tissues and helps you maintain your lean muscle mass. I don't know about you, but I really like my lean muscle mass (it burns more calories than fat).

I don't want anyone to stop eating protein, but certain proteins — such as beef — are far more acid-forming in your digestive tract than say, chicken. The following list shows the meat sources to avoid ranked from bad to worst:

- **Least acid forming:** Chicken, cold-water fish, duck, goose, shellfish

- **Moderately acid forming:** Lamb, pork, mussels, farmed fish, and wild game — elk, wild turkey, venison

- **Very acid forming:** Beef, lobster, organ meats (such as liver and kidney), smoked or processed meats

Potatoes — the fake veggie?

I hate to say it, but white potatoes are more akin to a snack food than a vegetable. This has to do with a little something called the *glycemic index*, which is the measurement of a food's impact on your blood sugar. Your body breaks all carbohydrates down into sugar for energy, but some are broken down more quickly than others.

The more complex a carbohydrate is, the longer it takes your body to break it down (and the lower number it gets assigned on the glycemic index). White potatoes fall under the heading of starches, which are basically simple sugars (and have a very high glycemic index).

The spuds start their digestive journey in your mouth as the enzymes in your saliva start to attack the simple sugar. It doesn't take very long for the potato to hit your blood stream in the form of sugar, which eventually causes an energy dive as your body goes into "clean up on aisle 6 mode" and tries to dump the sugars from your bloodstream.

So, instead of baking those tubers this weekend, try some sweet potatoes instead. These orange root veggies have all the fiber, vitamins, and minerals and fewer simple sugars than their white cousin.

Getting a grip on grains, nuts, and oils

You hear enough on the news about how certain grains protect your heart and can even lower your cholesterol, but did you know that some are acid-forming? Same thing goes for those delicious nuts and oils. Remember, nuts and oils are largely composed of fat and should be used sparingly in any diet, not just a pH balanced one.

The top acid-forming grains, nuts, and oils to limit or avoid altogether include

- ✔ **Least acid forming:** Brown rice, buckwheat, canola oil, pecans, processed oats
- ✔ **Moderately acid forming:** Corn oil, groats, palm kernel oil, peanut oil, rye, safflower oil, sesame oil
- ✔ **Very acid forming:** Brazil nuts, cashews, hazelnuts, pistachios, wheat and all its derivatives — including bread, flour, and pasta — wheat germ, white rice

Milking the dairy

True dairy products are inescapably animal products. It doesn't matter if you're snacking on a chunk of cheese or drinking a glass of skimmed milk — they both came from a cow.

Animal products in any form are acid-forming in our bodies. Consider the variety of acidifying dairy products to avoid:

- **Least acid forming:** Butter, goat cheese, yogurt

- **Moderately acid forming:** Goat milk, margarine, sheep's milk

- **Very acid forming:** *Casein* (milk protein derivative), cow milk, cream, egg yolk, processed cheese

Calling all other acid-formers

Despite all the lists in the preceding sections, there are still a number of beverages, preservatives, and other substances that form acid in your body. Most of these hidden acidifiers are used to cook or flavor food. Just imagine — when was the last time you had a spoonful of yeast? (I think I just threw up a little.)

The following list provides many of the hidden culinary ingredients that may tip an otherwise healthy, pH-balanced meal into acidity.

- **Least acid forming:** Gelatin, honey (processed honey, not clover honey), syrup, tea, distilled vinegar, rice vinegar

- **Moderately acid forming:** Coffee, vanilla, balsamic vinegar

- **Very acid forming:** Alcohol, artificial sweeteners, cocoa, condiments (the worst include ketchup, mayonnaise, and pickle relish), hops, soft drinks, sugar (brown, white, and confectioners), yeast

Keep in mind that I cannot possibly list every food, drink, and condiment that contains acidifying ingredients. If you have a bottle of ketchup lying around, take a peek at the label. Dollars to donuts it lists two acid-forming no-no's:

- Corn syrup

- Distilled vinegar

Almost every canned, jarred, or processed food has a label. Read the label and focus on the ingredient list. If it lists more preservatives and sugar than it does natural contents, chances are it's acid-forming.

Getting the Skinny on Sulfites

If you're one of the poor souls allergic to this compound, then you know that a sensitivity to sulfites cuts a whole lot of foods from your grocery list.

Sulfites are a chemical compound that occur naturally in fermented foods (beer, wine) or are added artificially to retain a food's color and texture, such as in a can of potatoes.

So what? About 1 out of every 100 people has a sulfite sensitivity. Sulfite sensitivities can turn into a full-blown allergy and cause anything from an itchy set of hives to a swollen-shut throat. Not to mention, the sulfite compound ranks about a negative 2.0 on the pH scale (acid!), so pretty much any food or drink containing sulfites is going to make your pH drop into acid-land.

Preserving foods

Face the facts: A tomato should not have a shelf life of ten years. But if you stick them in a can and preserve them, they'll stay a pretty bright red and still taste about the same a decade from now. It's the sulfites that make this possible. The next time you pick up a processed box, can, or tin of anything, check to see if sulfites are listed as an ingredient in the preserving process.

Banning the use

If you or a loved one has a true sulfite allergy, eating a food with this compound can elicit a potentially life-threatening response. Because of this, the use of sulfites on fresh fruits and vegetables (the ready-to-eat kind) has been banned in most countries.

It's still smart to give ready-to-eat products a thorough washing, just in case.

Identifying hidden sources

Although it's not an all-inclusive list, Table 11-1 shows some of the biggest sulfite-offenders. When in doubt (or definitely if you are cooking for someone who has a sulfite allergy), read the label.

Most governments now insist that any food containing more than ten parts per million (PPM) sulfites must list it in the ingredients.

Table 11-1		Foods Commonly Containing Sulfites		
Vegetables	*Fruits*	*Baked Goods*	*Beverages*	*Condiments*
Canned	Canned	Batters	Beer	Horseradish
Juices	Cider	Crackers	Canned drinks	Red wine vinegar
Pickled or commercially made	Jam	Flour tortillas	Instant tea mix	Relishes
	Juice	Pizza dough	Wine	Salad dressings
	Pie filling			

Pairing Foods Wisely

Even though I wouldn't encourage it, if you pair four ounces of red meat with a huge glass of lemon water, the acidifying effect of the red meat is somewhat negated by the lemon water. It's that yin and yang principle — the alkaline-forming ash of the lemon helps to combat the acid-forming ash of the meat. Having said that, you probably won't ever see a healthy alkaline pH result from this method — you just won't be doing quite as much damage to your body.

Creating the perfect match

When you make up your dinner plate tonight, plan to cover at least three-quarters of it in alkaline-forming foods. The remaining acids can consist of whatever delights your palate, but pick from the least acid-forming foods for the most pH benefit.

I like to think of it as eating a rainbow. Oh, I know it sounds corny, but it works in my kitchen. If we have a bland-colored protein (think tofu), I like to pair it with some vibrant green spinach, red peppers, and steamed carrots.

Paying attention to synergy

You have three digestive organs that produce enzymatic juices to break down food including your

- Stomach
- Pancreas
- Liver

Each organ plays a part in breaking down protein, carbohydrates, and fat to their absorbable parts, although these three food types are not broken down at the same rate.

Carbohydrates are dissolved the fastest, followed by protein, then fat. Fats stay in your stomach the longest, so it's wise to modulate the amount of fats you eat at each meal. Otherwise, foods can stagnate in your digestive tract waiting for the fat to be processed.

If that doesn't sound important, think about how lovely your sink would smell after a day if the drain were plugged. Bacteria starts to grow like it's on steroids and your flatulence (toots, farting, whatever you call it) will skyrocket.

Besides worrying about the intestinal orchestra, vitamins require a specific medium — either water or fat — to dissolve and be properly absorbed in your intestines. The fat-soluble vitamins are:

- Vitamin A
- Vitamin E
- Vitamin D
- Vitamin K

These four vitamins require some amount of fat for digestion, which is usually supplied naturally with your food. That probably explains why calcium and vitamin D are absorbed so well by simply drinking cow's milk — it has plenty of fat. Don't be fooled; you still ingest fats on an acid alkaline diet, but they're healthy fats, not artery-clogging ones.

The two water-soluble vitamins, vitamin C and the B family, dissolve simply with a little bit of fluid. Your body cannot store water-soluble vitamins, so it needs a fresh supply daily. Chances are, if you're eating a well-balanced diet, you're getting the nutrients your body needs to survive.

Chapter 12

Supplements, and Drinks, and Pills (Oh, My!)

*J*ust because you live in an era when you can drink the majority of your meals doesn't mean that liquid nutrients are the best choice for pH balance. In this chapter, I review how seemingly innocuous things like workout supplements or convenient meal-replacement shakes have the potential to increase your acidity.

Everything that passes your lips (ends up on your hips — okay, okay, just kidding) has the potential to increase or decrease your cellular pH. This chapter delves into the nitty-gritty territory of prescription and over-the-counter medications, supplements, and workout-enhancing drugs.

This chapter also addresses a million-dollar industry: enhanced drinking waters and dietary fiber supplements. You need both water and fiber, of course, because without water you would shortly be dead, and without fiber your time on the toilet could be real uncomfortable. But you can probably can get along just fine without that super-expensive bottle of water or gummy fiber supplement.

Are generic drugs acid-forming?

Generic is the term given to prescription or over-the-counter medications that are bioequivalent to the brand name drug. The manufacturers are bound by law to make sure the generic drug's active ingredient has the same potency and works the same as the brand name version. For instance, acetaminophen has the same active ingredient as the brand name Tylenol, just as ibuprofen has the same medication as its brand name counterpart Motrin. Acetaminophen and ibuprofen are considered generic versions of Tylenol and Motrin.

Regardless of whether the medicine you take is purchased over the counter or by prescription only, many common medications have a generic counterpart. The generic version is usually less expensive and it's sometimes the only one covered by an insurance prescription plan.

The portion of the generic drug that may not be the exact same as its brand name counterpart is the *excipients*, or the inactive ingredients in the medication. These can include things like the dyes used to color it, the binding agents, or the fillers. These extra ingredients may contain substances like cornstarch, lactose, sucrose, or even gelatin, all of which are acid-forming in your body.

Hypothetically, the excipients have the potential to change the way your body uses a medication. This is the main reason why some people state they cannot use a generic version of a drug, as it may not elicit the same effect as the brand name offered. Talk to your doctor if you're taking a generic drug and have concerns about its performance or effects in your body.

Popping Pills and Altering Your pH

A pain reliever here, a meal replacement there . . . what harm can they really do to your pH? Unfortunately, no large studies have been carried out on this topic. What I can tell you is that some of the easily accessible so-called health supplements may not be what they seem on the surface.

In this section, I help you identify the supplements, shakes, and even pills that can negatively impact your pH. In other chapters I mention the fact that worry, lack of sleep, and even prolonged stress can acidify you; now I'm going to add to the list — every single thing you put in your mouth potentially impacts your pH balance.

Talk to your doctor before altering your medications, including over-the-counter, herbal, or especially prescription drugs. He or she can discuss any concerns you have. I'm not a doctor and I don't play one on TV, so don't ask me about them. I'm just here to inform you that some drugs can and do affect your pH balance.

Getting a grip on over-the-counter pills

You can buy it without a prescription, so it has to be safe, right? Wrong. What's safe for you may not be safe for me and vice versa. Certain over-the-counter (OTC) drugs can make your pH fluctuate. Before you do the happy dance when you see a morning urine pH of 7.5, take into consideration the OTC drugs that can zip your pH right up the scale into alkaline territory.

And before you say, "Who cares what caused it — isn't it great that my pH is alkaline now?" I'll remind you that it's an artificial bump into alkalinity caused by the OTC medications.

A high pH reading after taking certain medications may only mean that your urine is flushing out the alkaline medications, not that your tissues are becoming more alkaline. That's like those underpants that make your bottom look sculpted, but the effect comes from special padding, not buns of steel. It's false advertising. Don't depend on urine pH results for a day or two after taking:

- Alka-Seltzer, Amphojel
- Baking soda (some people still use it as a home remedy for heartburn)
- Calcium supplements
- Echinacea
- Gaviscon
- Maalox, Mylanta
- Magnesium
- Milk of magnesia
- Mineral supplementation
- Pepto-Bismol, Rolaids
- Sea kelp supplements
- TUMS
- Valerian root

Scientific research and trials are resulting in new OTC formulas daily, so it's impossible to create an all-inclusive list of drugs that impact your pH. However, now you know some that can!

Treading carefully: Prescription drugs

Certain prescription drugs have the capability of altering your pH — especially the ones that deal with your fluid levels, electrolytes, and mineral absorption. Electrolytes are charged ions — they conduct electricity throughout your body, which allows your cells to communicate with one another. Specifically, the minerals potassium, calcium, and sodium, which become electrolytes within your body, play huge roles in your pH balancing mechanisms.

Your fluid and electrolytes are intricately tied to your pH balance. It's the minerals remaining in the alkaline ash of foods that correct your pH. Flush out those alkaline minerals and watch your pH become acidic. (Same thing can happen with prolonged vomiting or diarrhea.) The prescription drugs most closely associated with your pH balance include:

- **Furosemide** and **hydrochlorothiazide** (say that three times fast) are usually prescribed to help treat cardiovascular disorders such as congestive heart failure (CHF) or high blood pressure and swelling (fluid retention) due to kidney or liver failure. Known as *potassium-wasting diuretics,* basically, they make you pee to flush out unnecessary fluids. However, these drugs also cause you to lose valuable electrolytes including potassium, sodium, and chloride, all of which may impact your pH.

- **Potassium supplements,** even though you can buy them over the counter, should be used only if your doctor recommends it. They're usually prescribed for people who take diuretics to compensate for the electrolyte loss. Too little of this electrolyte in your body and your muscles can become weak and your heartbeat may become irregular. The majority of people get enough potassium by eating healthy foods including spinach and lentils.

Research is showing that the active ingredient in black licorice, glycyrrhizic acid, has the potential to dump potassium out of your body as well.

If your doctor has told you to bump up the potassium and minerals in your diet by natural means, you're in luck, and your pH balance is fortunate as well. Many fruits and vegetables on the acid alkaline diet are potassium rich. Consider eating more:

- Avocadoes
- Bananas
- Lentils
- Mangos

✔ Oranges and fresh-squeezed orange juice

✔ Spinach

✔ Sweet potatoes

✔ Tomatoes

Examining the Price You Pay for Getting Ripped

If you want six-pack abs, bulging deltoids, rock hard thighs, and you want them by next week, keep dreaming. Fact is, your body's just not made that way. Lean muscle mass is built through a process of stretching and straining current muscle fibers until they form a new, thicker layer. You probably won't see the ripped muscular physique you dream of for months — maybe even longer depending on how much fluff lies over those muscles.

This information may come as a surprise to you having been bombarded with ads for workout and bodybuilding supplements that claim you can have the body you dream of in mere weeks.

Trimming workout supplements

I'll put this out on the table now: I'm not a huge fan of pumping my body full of creatine, caffeine, testosterone, or diuretics. In some form, each and every one of these substances may be hiding in that pill or drink you're using in hopes of getting ripped a little faster.

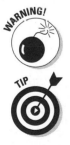

I won't even mention steroids (anabolic or designer), because they're illegal in most places and harm your health in innumerable ways.

If you're using workout supplements, take the time to read the label and learn about what you're putting into your body, which may include the following:

✔ **Caffeine** is considered a safe pick-me-up at levels less than 400 milligrams per day, or a couple small cups of coffee. However, as I mention, caffeine is acid-forming in your body. Make sure to check the serving size — the manufacturer may list the amount of caffeine contained in one scoop of supplement or one pill, but encourage you to take two to four on the dosage instructions. You may also want to consider how much daily caffeine you get outside of the workout supplement.

Too much caffeine can cause nervousness, irritation, and insomnia among other uncomfortable side effects.

✔ **Creatine** is probably one of the most popular workout supplements. It's used to improve athletic performance by stimulating the muscles to release energy more quickly. Your body already makes creatine in your liver, stores it in the muscles, and it's also supplied through your diet. If you're taking large amounts of creatine, chances are your kidneys are filtering out the excess (giving you really expensive pee and nothing else).

✔ **Diuretics** are drugs or supplements (caffeine) that make you urinate more, which causes your kidneys to flush out alkalinizing minerals with the pee.

Diuretics in workout supplements can be dangerous. They force your body into a state of dehydration, which overworks your kidneys, ruins your electrolyte balance, and can lead to heart *arrythmias* (wonky heart beat). Athletes may use them to temporarily decrease their weight (known as *cutting*) and temporarily improve performance, but this practice is highly discouraged by the medical community. If you want to naturally drop a little water weight and stay alkaline, eat a slice of watermelon.

✔ **Testosterone** is a naturally occurring hormone in both men and women, although women have far less. This hormone powers the male sexual and gender characteristics (deep voice, muscle mass) and is commercially promoted to help build bulky muscles. A number of workout supplements contain testosterone-enhancing agents, either chemical concoctions or herbal supplements to stimulate production of the hormone.

Stimulating your body to make excess testosterone without an actual deficiency can have a number of ill effects in both genders. Men can suffer an enlarged prostate, decreased sperm count, acne, and breast growth. Women may get a deeper voice, facial hair, and an enlarged clitoris.

Health bars and shakes

Health bars, such as protein snack bars, and shakes may have their place in a well-balanced diet, but you have to know what to look for in a quality product. Many of the bars marketed as a healthy meal replacement or a post-workout snack are also chalk full of calories, fat, and other questionable ingredients that can acidify your pH.

Do you really need a recovery drink?

Science and nutrition experts have been battling over the best recovery drink formula for years. A *recovery drink* is used to replenish depleted muscles after an intense workout. It is not the same thing as a sports drink, which usually contains electrolytes (and sometimes large amounts of sugar) to rehydrate your body after exercise.

Experts have found that a well-balanced recovery drink needs a 2:1 ratio of carbohydrates and proteins to properly stimulate muscle recovery. The amino acids (small building blocks of protein), specifically one called leucine, boost your insulin performance and assist protein metabolism. The carbohydrates refuel the depleted glycogen (sugar) stores in your muscles. Together, the protein and carbohydrates help your muscle fibers grow stronger resulting in increased lean muscle mass.

Without the proper nutrition following a hard workout, you may start to show signs of poor muscle recovery including:

✔ Fatigue (prolonged after your workout)

✔ Excessive muscle soreness

✔ Decreasing strength (should be increasing)

✔ An inability to grow lean muscle mass

If you decide to use a recovery drink but are worried about your pH impact, you can make one at home without any fillers or chemicals. Mix six ounces of fresh squeezed fruit juice (carbohydrates) with a scoop of whey protein powder (protein) and you have a pH balanced recovery drink. Just be sure to drink it within two hours following the exercise session, as this is when your body is primed to shuttle the nutrients to your warm muscles.

Ask the following questions about bars and shakes before buying them:

✔ **Why is the product is appealing to you?** Is it the convenience? Taste? Promise of weight loss? All of these things can be accomplished with a healthy acid alkaline balanced meal without the high price tag usually associated with convenience health foods.

✔ **Does the product meet your dietary needs?** Make sure the product has sufficient calories, vitamins, minerals, protein, and fiber to meet your needs — especially if you're using the bar or shake as a meal replacement. A protein bar containing 20 grams of protein and not much else is not a meal replacement; it's a high-protein snack.

Adult protein requirements vary by body size, health, and activity level, but the average adult only needs between 30 and 60 grams per day (these recommendations vary widely, obviously). When it's not used to rebuild lean muscle mass or heal your tissues, excess protein becomes fat.

✔ **Do you feel full after eating it?** I've tried a couple meal replacement shake systems and gained weight. I was so hungry 15 minutes after consuming the shakes that I ended up eating twice as many calories on the program as I did before trying to drink the meal replacements. You can try what I did, and drink a big glass of water to trick your stomach that it's full, but the effect doesn't last too long.

✔ **What are the ingredients?** Just like other prepackaged products, some meal and snack bars have acid-forming fillers. Look for the hidden sugars, acid-forming grains, and preservatives. Many shake-type meal replacements contain casein, an acid-forming milk protein.

Your best pH bet is to find one that contains whey protein, which is not acid-forming during digestion.

Debunking the Beverage Hype

Alkalinizing drinks, sports drinks, recovery drinks . . . so many commercialized choices and so little time. Hopefully, after reading this section, you'll become a savvier beverage consumer (and maybe even save a little cash). Think twice about what liquid you choose to fill up your cup; just like food, beverages can make or break your pH.

Many experts recommend drinking half your weight in ounces of water daily for optimum hydration. According to that formula, a 100-pound person should be drinking at least 50 ounces of water daily for health. If you exercise, spend time in a warm climate, or drink liquids that make you urinate more frequently (caffeinated beverages, alcohol), you need to drink even more water.

Oxygenated water

I found a $500 machine online that oxygenates your water to "make it more healthy." Water is a colorless, odorless, tasteless compound that can be a liquid, gas, or solid. It's sometimes called by its chemical name: H_2O, which stands for *dihydrogen* (two hydrogen molecules) *monoxide* (one oxygen molecule). If you add more oxygen molecules to it, won't it become H_2O_2? That's the chemical name for hydrogen peroxide, which you shouldn't drink.

Although I'm no chemist, a water molecule is a water molecule. If you try to alter the chemical composition of the molecule in any way, it becomes something else (like hydrogen peroxide). Some of these water oxygenating machines claim to vigorously swirl water to incorporate more oxygen molecules. Personally, I'll save my money under the mattress and vigorously shake my glass of water instead.

Examining alkaline water

Half the people you talk to state that drinking alkaline water to improve pH is a hoax, the other half say it benefits their pH and health tremendously. I can give you the premise, but scientific research on this topic is sadly scarce.

Although they are difficult to find in the grocery store or corner market, several manufacturers sell bottled alkaline water. Some brand names I've found, ranging from the most to the least expensive, include Essentia, Alkazone, and Alka Pure.

The cheapest way to boost the alkaline component in your plain water is by adding fresh squeezed lemon or lime juice. The minerals in the juice leave an alkaline ash after the water is absorbed. This doesn't technically make the water alkaline, but it does increase its alkaline-forming potential. Drink the lemon water through a straw and save your tooth enamel.

Your best bet after making your own or using an ionizer (see the upcoming "Ionizers" section), you can purchase alkaline water at the store. If it isn't labeled alkaline water, look for the key buzzwords of *microwater, ionized water, micro-clustered water,* or *real mineral water* (not created, but bottled at the source).

Don't take any medications with alkaline water. In theory, true alkaline water has smaller molecules that can increase the absorption of medicine and enhance its effects (not in a good way). To be on the safe side, discuss the ramifications of drinking alkaline water with your doctor, and ask how long you should wait to drink it before and after taking your medicine.

The following sections explore the different ways people make their drinking water more alkaline.

Alkaline water filters

If you see a claim for an alkaline water filter, run in the opposite direction from this blatant misrepresentation. Filtering water removes some of the things like pesticides, heavy metals, and chemicals used during processing. But a water filter, whether it attaches to your sink or sits in a pretty little canister, cannot make alkaline water.

Some experts argue that filtered water actually has a lower pH (acidic) than tap water. Having said that, I wouldn't drink tap water without a filter. Know your water source whether it's city water, well water, or from another source, and request a quality test if you have concerns about your tap water.

Alkaline water drops

Many different manufacturers promote and sell pH-balancing drops for water. The claim is that these drops add minerals to the water and increase the overall pH (sounds kind of like adding fresh-squeezed lemon juice to the water for the alkalinizing minerals, but what do I know).

If you chose to use pH drops, always follow the manufacturer's recommendations and warnings. I've tried some of these — a few gave the water a bitter taste. See whether you can try samples before committing to a purchase.

Ionizers

As far as I'm aware, the one true way to alkalinize water is with an ionizing machine. They are costly, but they deliver pure, filtered alkaline water with an average pH between 9.5 and 10 (some models even let you control the level of alkalinity). The majority of models come equipped with a filtration system, so you also need to pay for new filters as needed.

Microwater

Ionizing advocates claim that the process breaks down water molecules and makes them smaller, which in theory is easier to digest, absorb, and transport throughout your body. The tiny molecules of water are sometimes called *microwater* or *micro-clustered* water.

Suffering sports drinks

With two busy young boys, I know all about the need to replenish fluids and electrolytes after nine innings of baseball in 92-degree weather. But I sure don't want to pump their bodies full of sugar, too!

Check the label on your commercial sports drink. You don't want it to contain grams of sugar or artificial sweeteners, which boost the calorie content and form acids, not rehydrate you. What you want instead are some important electrolytes, such as:

- Calcium
- Magnesium
- Phosphate
- Potassium
- Sodium

Vetting vitamin enhanced waters

I can add vitamins to a cheeseburger, but that still won't make it my best nutritional option. Likewise, I could sprinkle some vitamin C and powdered fiber in a glass of red wine, but it's still not a health drink (don't even think about it).

If you opt to purchase one of the vitamin-enhanced beverages out there, you may want to consider the label carefully. The majority of the ones I've seen contain either whole sugar or an acid-forming artificial sweetener.

If you're eating a pH balanced diet, chances are you're getting enough vitamins in their natural form. However, if you're worried about a vitamin deficiency, talk to your doctor; he or she can point you in the direction of a daily multiple vitamin to meet your needs.

One more thing to think about: Most vitamin-enhanced beverages contain the water-soluble vitamins B and C. Your body can only use so much of these vitamins daily; it cannot store excess. If you're overloading on vitamins B and C, the majority of them are probably getting filtered out of your body and making your pee really rich in vitamins, which does nothing but flush money down the toilet (literally).

Energizing drinks

Energizing commercial drinks come in many different forms including the obvious stimulating drinks to the less-obvious flavored calorie-free water-enhancing drops.

If a drink lists caffeine as an ingredient, it's acid-forming and should be limited or avoided altogether on a pH balanced diet. If you haven't already checked out Chapter 6, now would be a good time. I talk all about caffeine and the acid-forming effect of this stimulant in that chapter.

When you feel the need an afternoon pick-me-up, consider taking a quick break and going for a walk. Let the exercise and fresh air rejuvenate you! A healthy snack may also do the trick — your blood sugar could take a dip in the hours after lunch, which can make you feel tired and irritable. Munch on some almonds or fresh fruit to bring your blood sugar back up.

Ouch! Dealing with hemorrhoids

Hemorrhoids may be the butt of many jokes (no pun intended), but if you've ever experienced them, they aren't funny. *Hemorrhoid* is the preferred name given to swollen veins around your anus. They can be internal (on the inside) or external (on the outside) and cause severe discomfort and itching in your bum. Some of the veins can bleed, leaving you to worry about the bright red blood on your toilet paper.

One of the best ways to help prevent hemorrhoids is by eating a diet high in fiber and drinking plenty of water. When you sit on the toilet and strain (or read a newspaper), these veins become engorged with blood. Some hemorrhoids go away on their own, but others may need surgical removal, which doesn't sound like a lot of fun to me.

You can decrease your discomfort at home by:

✔ Soaking your bum in warm water for 10 to 15 minutes (known as a sitz bath).

✔ Using over-the-counter preparation creams to reduce itching and discomfort.

✔ Wearing cotton underpants, which helps decrease moisture (synthetics hold onto moisture) around the hemorrhoids and helps with irritation.

✔ Using baby wipes or moist disposable wipes as opposed to toilet paper.

✔ Increasing the natural fiber in your diet.

✔ Using stool softeners to loosen hard stools and prevent straining during a bowel movement.

If you have anal discomfort, itching, or blood on your toilet paper, consult with your physician. He or she can confirm a suspicion of hemorrhoids and alleviate any concerns about more serious conditions that can lead to rectal bleeding, such as rectal or colon cancer.

Filling Up on Fiber

Fiber, roughage, cardboard (ha, ha) — whatever name you give it, *fiber* is the indigestible part of plant food. In and of itself, fiber is pH neutral, but its many health benefits within your body can work collaboratively to boost an acidic pH.

According to studies, most of us don't get enough fiber in our daily diet. Experts recommend aiming for 20 to 35 grams of the stuff as part of a healthy diet daily (more or less, depending on your age, mobility, and health). Seeing as how most fiber supplements offer between two to five grams of fiber, you may want to re-examine your fiber source. That fiber chewie may provide as little as ten percent of your daily fiber needs.

Plant foods contain two types of fiber:

- **Soluble:** As the names suggest, soluble fiber dissolves in water and acts like a big sponge sucking up fluids and slowing down digestion.

- **Insoluble:** Again, as the name implies, insoluble fiber does not dissolve — quite frankly, it doesn't even change that much passing through your digestive tract. Insoluble fiber gets the stool moving through your bowels like a big freight train.

The two types of fiber work together in your system. As long as you eat a varied, healthy diet, you're probably getting enough of both.

Taking supplements versus the real deal

Powders, pills, baked goods, cereals, gummy supplements, and now even enhanced artificial sweeteners are marketed to provide a source of quick fiber. With the commercialization of fiber's health benefits, it's no wonder part of the message got lost in the translation: It's not just the fiber that's good for you, it's the food source that provides it!

I have a true or false statement for you to ponder:

> As long as you consume at least 20 grams of fiber daily, it doesn't matter where it comes from.

False. Many of the health benefits of fiber stem from the fact that it's a part of a healthy, balanced diet — the naturally fibrous foods are filling, low calorie, and an important source of vitamins and minerals.

In fact, some experts argue that taking too much fiber in supplement form can actually rob your body of vitamins and minerals. As it travels through your digestive tract, the fake fiber can suck up and transport out many of the minerals that would've helped to alkalinize your body.

There are times when fiber supplements are a perfectly acceptable accompaniment to a healthy diet. You may need to take daily fiber supplements if you have:

- Been encouraged to do so by your doctor
- Certain intestinal disorders such as irritable bowel syndrome (IBS)
- Constipation while using prescription narcotics
- Chronic hemorrhoids
- Disorders that affect your digestive *motility* (how fast stool moves through your intestines)

Although you can take too much fiber in supplement form, you cannot technically overdose on fiber if you are eating it natural from whole foods.

Finding fiber

Check out your local produce stand — it's brimming with fiber. Most fruits and vegetables contain a mixture of soluble and insoluble fiber, so it's best to eat the entire fruit or vegetable (the skin and meat) if it's consumable. The edible skins of fruits and vegetables usually provide the insoluble fiber, whereas the softer meat inside is soluble.

To increase the insoluble fiber in your diet you can eat more:

- Edible fruit skins (apples, pears, peaches, apricots)
- Nuts (almonds)
- Vegetables (and edible skins, like sweet potatoes)

To increase the soluble fibers in your diet try adding:

- Beans, legumes
- Oats, barley
- Vegetables and fruit

Eat the foods as close to their natural (raw) form as possible. Overcooking fruits, vegetables, and grains decreases not only the fresh enzymes, vitamins, and minerals of the food, but it can also start to break down the fiber content.

Monitoring the effects in the body

It's a well-known fact that fiber improves the health of your colon, but this plant product has many other healthful purposes. Fiber can improve your cardiovascular and overall digestive health. For people with diabetes, this nutrient is emerging as a dietary staple for its effects on stabilizing blood sugar.

Increase your fiber intake slowly, as a rapid change in dietary fiber consumption may lead to:

- Painful bloating
- Diarrhea or constipation (also known as irregularity)
- Gas

It's a good idea to increase the amount of fluids you drink while increasing your fiber intake. Soluble fiber acts like a giant sponge, sucking up the fluid in your intestines. The upside — it makes for firmer, more regular, bulky stools. The downside — it can plug up your system really well if you don't drink enough water to flush it out.

Weight loss

Dollars to donuts, if you check out some popular weight loss supplements, they'll have some form of fiber listed as an active ingredient. Fiber is famous for making you feel full. The technical word for this is *satiety* — fiber expands and fills your stomach making you feel like you can't eat another bite and it lingers so that you won't want to eat again anytime soon.

Cardiovascular

Soluble fibers attach to fats in your bloodstream (cholesterol) and flush them out of your body. Decreased cholesterol levels can reduce your risk for high blood pressure, stroke, and heart attack.

Colon and digestive impacts

Soluble and insoluble fibers make your colon happy. They act like a broom and sweep out the excess garbage. The two types of fiber work together to regulate bowel movements; you don't want your stool too soft or frequent (diarrhea), and you don't want to strain on the toilet (constipation).

Fibrous foods also require a little more chewing action than simple sugars, which increases the digestion and absorption of nutrients. If you have to chew your food longer, chances are you eat it more slowly.

Diabetes

It's not groundbreaking news: A high-fiber diet can help regulate blood sugar. The fibers slow down the digestion of nutrients, which helps to reduce blood sugar fluctuations that can make you feel crummy. High-fiber foods are usually filling and low in calories, so they can help you manage your diet and help prevent overeating.

Part IV
Let's Eat!

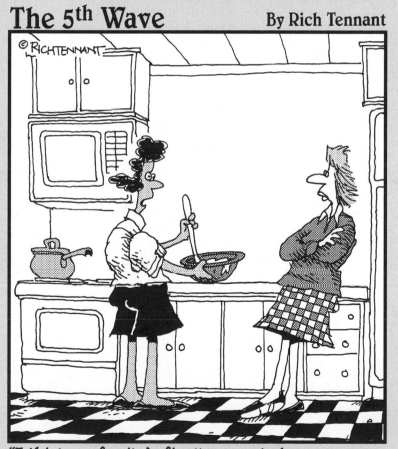

The 5th Wave   By Rich Tennant

"I think my family's finally accepted my new way
of cooking. I've eliminated all of the meat,
some of the fat, and most of the sarcasm."

In this part...

1 don't blame you if you skipped right to this part. It's wise to check out recipes and grocery lists before committing to a diet — you need to know what you're in for. I've got great news for you skip-aheaders: There's nothing weird or otherworldly about the acid alkaline diet. The grocery lists and recipes in this part contain many recognizable (and deliciously edible) foods, some of which you probably have on hand already. And believe me, if I can make these recipes, so can you.

Chapter 13

Making a List, Checking It Twice

Recipes in This Chapter

▶ Clarified Butter

This chapter covers my favorite arena: food! Before you start whipping up pH-happy meals, you need to mentally and physically prepare. Otherwise, what's going to happen? Your son's soccer game will run long and you'll be sticking a frozen meat lover's pizza in the oven, ruining your pH plans. Proper preparation helps you start on the right foot.

I've prepared a list of suggestions to help your meal planning (right down to the spices) so you can spend more time with the tykes or socializing, and less time figuring out what to eat. Use your smartphone to take pictures of spice lists or meal plans; that's why I typed them, so you don't have to.

I am not a professional chef. Grocery list exchanges are welcome — as long as you pay attention to the foods discussed in Chapter 11. I tend to like things a bit spicy (food and life); you can leave the spices off your shopping list if you have delicate taste buds.

Getting Ready Mentally

Repeat after me: "I am not trying out a fad diet to lose weight quickly. I am embarking on a healthy lifestyle change to improve my wellbeing." Make this your mantra over the next weeks, months — however long it takes you to fully transition to an acid alkaline lifestyle.

I am not fond of the word "diet." I think it has a negative connotation as something you *have to do* and adhere to. Although this book is titled, *Acid Alkaline Diet For Dummies*, I would have preferred *Acid Alkaline pH Balancing and Your Health and Well-Being For Dummies* (but that's a mouthful).

To tell or not to tell, that is the question

When I embarked on a vegan lifestyle a few years ago, I decided not to share it with anyone except my husband. I didn't hang a sign around my neck or vehemently refuse to eat meat — I just stopped. One beautiful aspect of the acid alkaline diet is that you don't have to tell anyone you're doing it, unless you want to. It's not an ostentatious diet — you won't be hiding pre-manufactured trays of food in the freezer or suddenly downing whole chickens but no biscuits. You just appear to be an extremely smart, nutritionally educated person when you are eating carrot sticks in lieu of cheese doodles.

If I may make one suggestion about people you should tell: Your family or the people you live with. Don't surprise them with the sudden exchange of "non-meat crumbles" for real hamburger on spaghetti night — it doesn't have a happy ending (trust me on that). And, if it suits you, consider discussing your choice with your friends — you may make a difference in their health and well-being.

Setting a start date

There are two schools of thought on how to start a new eating system:

- ✔ You can jump in with both feet and submerge yourself in the acid alkaline diet.
- ✔ You can slowly incorporate healthier choices over time.

I can't tell you what method to choose (you know yourself better than I do). I *can* tell you that it's easier to backslide (or never fully transition) if you go too slowly. It's human nature to put off your start date until tomorrow, next week, then the week after . . . get my drift?

I encourage taking baby steps toward your dietary goals throughout this book; however, it's scientifically proven that people who make changes cold turkey — they just quit eating acid-forming foods and don't slowly wean them out — have a better chance of success. Consider picking a start date and sticking with it. Complete this sentence: I will abandon an acid-forming lifestyle and start eating healthy, alkaline forming foods on (insert date here). Good for you! You just took the first step toward a healthier lifestyle!

Don't set yourself up for failure by setting a start date around holidays or special events, when adhering to any diet can be trickier. Pick a date, preferably two to three weeks from today, when you will start your diet or begin incorporating healthier pH food choices. This should give you enough time to gather supplies (if you want to use the pH testing strips discussed in Chapter 4), and food and to start experimenting with recipes.

Realizing it's not a trend, it's a lifestyle

I've said it before and I'll say it again. Balancing your pH is not a trend or a fad. You won't be doing anything crazy or weird (well, except for maybe dipping litmus strips in your urine) like eating hoards of protein, baby food, or taking coffee enemas. You *will* be changing the way you approach what you eat and drink, lessening your body's workload, and flushing out years of acid stored in your cells.

If recent attempts at dietary improvement have failed, set yourself up for success by:

- ✔ Examining *why* past attempts failed (time, money, commitment)
- ✔ Involving loved ones in your plan
- ✔ Setting goals and sticking to them
- ✔ Making one lifestyle change at a time

That last one is a biggie. If you try to do everything at once — stop smoking, quit drinking alcohol, drop red meat from your diet, and so on — your chances of failing to make any change increase. Instead, consider setting short-term goals for each lifestyle factor you would like to change: "Next week, I'll start a smoking cessation class. The following week, I'll replace red meat with fish." As a good friend once told me, "You can't eat a rhinoceros in one bite" (although I'm not sure who would want to). However, you can overcome any task if you break it down into smaller pieces.

Making Food Selections

Most grocery stores are set up the same way: Produce and natural products are placed around the perimeter of the store, canned goods, boxed dinners, and prepackaged meals are placed in the aisles.

Spend *more time* shopping around the perimeter of the store and *less time* perusing prepackaged and convenience foods in the aisles. Better yet, hit the local farmer's market and pick up fruits and vegetables that are in season. These are usually less expensive and will keep you away from the convenience-type foods, which can be acidifying.

Reading the label

Prepackaged foods contain a nutritional label. Although the looks of the label will vary by your geographical region, the contents are pretty much the same:

- ✔ **Serving size:** The recommended portion size (usually not the whole container of food unless it is marked "single serving").

- ✔ **Calories:** The amount of energy in the food.

- ✔ **Calories from fat:** How much of that energy comes from an unhealthy source.

- ✔ **Total fat:** You need fat to live, but not the saturated fat in prepackaged foods — that's the heart-attack and stroke-causing kind. Check out Chapter 2 for more fat facts.

- ✔ **Saturated and trans fats:** The bad fats that you should avoid.

- ✔ **Cholesterol:** Lipid (fat) found in animal foods and produced by your liver. Excess cholesterol can lead to heart disease and stroke.

- ✔ **Sodium:** The fancy name for salt. People with cardiovascular or kidney disease may be on a sodium-restricted diet.

- ✔ **Carbohydrates:** A macronutrient you need to live; carbs include fiber and sugar.

- ✔ **Protein:** A macronutrient required for energy and tissue repair.

WARNING!

Take a long look at the list of ingredients before you buy a packaged food. Many prepackaged foods contain pH-affecting additives such as:

- ✔ Artificial sweeteners (acidifying)

- ✔ Baking soda (alkalinizing)

- ✔ Bleached flour (acidifying)

- ✔ Salt (alkalinizing)

If you're doing your best to adhere to an acid alkaline diet and your pH is still out of whack, you may be accidentally ingesting acidifying substances hidden in a convenience food — check your labels. When in doubt, cut the foods out for a bit and see if the problem resolves.

Selecting produce

Yep, it's okay to give a little squeeze to check for freshness. No one wants to pay for a rotten grapefruit. Because the bulk (about 80 percent) of your acid alkaline diet is composed of fruits and vegetables, you will become very adept at spotting an about-to-turn-bad eggplant or a canned vegetable with more sodium than nutrients.

The fresh kind

Overall, fresh produce is your best choice. Fresh fruits and vegetables have intact enzymes — catalysts that aid digestion and help your body absorb vitamins and nutrients. Heating and processing fresh produce kills the enzymes and leaches out some of the alkalinizing minerals.

Fresh fruits and vegetables should have:

- ✔ Bright colors
- ✔ No shriveling
- ✔ No soft or brown spots
- ✔ Shiny, tight skins

The frozen kind

You don't have to eat *everything* fresh. Plenty of fruits and vegetables found in the freezer section are still okay on an acid alkaline diet. But you have to know what to look for:

- ✔ Avoid fruits or vegetables with sauces; get the plain kind.
- ✔ Choose flash-frozen.
- ✔ Pick produce with no added ingredients, such as sugar or preservatives.

The canned kind

Running late at work and don't have time to hit the produce stand? That's okay. The biggest downside to a diet rich in plant foods is that they go bad fairly quickly. You can use the canned kind of fruits and vegetables, but be sure to check labels and know what you are purchasing.

Avoid canned foods with:

- ✔ Added sodium
- ✔ Ingredients other than the fruit or vegetable
- ✔ Syrup

I know they're cheaper, but avoid purchasing dented or compromised cans. The food in these cans is suspect at the least, and saturated with microbes (think botulism) at the worst. Also, be sure to rinse the fruits or vegetables after removing them from the can. This will help to wash off any preservatives (such as sodium).

Stocking up on spices

Spices can add sensational flavor and aroma to almost any dish. They bring out the natural flavors in cooked veggies, poultry, and fish, and they allow you to use less fatty oils for flavoring meats and other dishes.

Table 13-1 shows the herbs most suited to various foods:

Table 13-1	Spice-Food Pairings
Salads and Vegetables	***Chicken, Fish, and Other Meats***
Dill seeds	Basil
Garlic	Cayenne
Oregano	Curry powder
Rosemary	Dill
Sage	Garlic
Thyme	Marjoram
Fresh or Roasted Fruits	Onion powder
Allspice	Oregano
Cinnamon	Paprika
Cloves	Rosemary
Ginger	Thyme
Mint	
Nutmeg	

Drafting Weekly Grocery Lists

Want to spend more money than necessary and still come home without the proper ingredients to put together a savory meal? No, me either. Making a grocery list saves you unnecessary trips back and forth to the store and saves you money as well.

To make your shopping experience productive, use these tips:

✔ Don't shop when you're hungry. You're more susceptible to impulse purchases.

✔ Keep your list and coupons in your car, briefcase, or handbag so they're available when you need them.

✔ Leave the kids at home, if possible. Without these lovable distractions, you can take your time and focus on the task at hand.

Stop winging it

It only takes a few minutes to sit down and plan every meal for the family that week. Plan for the basics — breakfast, lunch, and dinner — and include snacks and foods for any special occasions coming up. Don't forget lunches for your children, your spouse, and lunches at work.

Of course, I have no idea what you intend to cook for dinner tonight or breakfast tomorrow. Table 13-2 shows a possible weekly menu using recipes from the hoards provided in Chapters 14 through 17.

Table 13-2		Weekly Meal Plan		
	Breakfast	**Lunch**	**Dinner**	**Snack or Dessert**
Monday	Grapefruit and Groovy Granola	Gazpacho	Stuffed Peppers	Kale Chips
Tuesday	Whey Good Smoothie	Spinach Medley	Veggie Bake	Holy Guacamole
Wednesday	Farmer's Omelet	Sweet N' Sour Salad	Eggplant Curry	Silky Lemon Pie
Thursday	Breakfast Scrambler	Hearty Chicken Soup	Salmon with Lemony Fettuccini	Better Baked Apples
Friday	Bananas for Oatmeal	Fresh Veggie Soup	Chicken Hash	Bagged Popcorn
Saturday	Asparagus Omelet	Zucchini Quesadillas	Pizza	Oatmeal Cookies
Sunday	EZ Curried Eggs	Chili	Stuffed Green Peppers	Scrumptious Salsa

While drafting your weekly meal plans, keep the 80-20 percentages in mind — 80 percent of your foods should be alkaline-forming, only 20 percent acidifying to maximize your pH balancing potential. You can eat acidifying foods, but your meals and grocery list should be heavy on the alkaline-forming foods. (For lists of what those are, check out Chapter 11.)

Now that I have your taste buds going, check out the recipes and see how many ingredients you already have on hand. Then, draft your grocery list and get shopping.

Spending your grocery money wisely

It's a sad fact — healthy diets cost more. But you can save your money for something fun (like a vacation) and stop wasting it at the grocery store. You don't have to go broke eating healthy foods, but you *do* have to learn how to shop wisely.

Buying what's in season

If you want a strawberry (very alkalinizing, by the way) in the middle of December, you are going to have to pay extra for that juicy fruit. Eating whatever crop is in season can save money and provides variation in your diet. I'm not a farmer, and chances are you aren't either. To find out more about seasonal produce in your geographical location:

✔ Ask a long-time resident.

✔ Check online.

✔ Visit farmers' markets and produce stands.

Checking the fliers

Small and large, most grocery stores produce weekly fliers touting their deals of the week and upcoming sales. If you don't find the fliers in your mail, check the weekly paper or ask a clerk at the store. You can also go online to your favorite establishment's website and find your location.

Using that smartphone

If you have one of the many different types of smartphones, you may not even have to clip coupons. Many phones have barcode apps or coupon apps that allow you to use the phone as your coupon collector.

Preparing Your Kitchen

Your refrigerator and pantry are now bursting at the seams with alkalinizing, healthy, pH-balancing foods, right? But you're not quite ready to get started cooking. (Don't you just hate that?)

Many of my recipes contain some ingredients that may be foreign to you. Before I became a pH'er, I didn't know much about these ingredients, either. However, they *can* make the difference between an acid-forming meal and an alkalinizing one. Take eggs, for example. Find me a baked good that doesn't include them. They're awesome! Eggs hold things together and help cakes get fluffy. But . . . they are also an animal protein, which leave an acid ash. I'm not saying you can't ever eat eggs again — I'm saying it's better, on a daily basis, to use egg substitutes or egg whites to maintain your pH balance.

The following sections talk about some tools and foods you should get used to.

Cooking paraphernalia

When I got married (many moons ago), I didn't know the difference between a sauté pan and a skillet. Confidentially, not much has changed. I don't have a collection of designer cookware, and you won't need one, either (but feel free to tell your spouse you do, if you're looking for new pots and pans). I pick the utensil, skillet, or dish that does the job.

Nonstick cookware is the only exception I make to the "don't need new cookware" rule. If you don't have any — invest. I don't get paid to sponsor or drop names, so I won't. Pick and choose whatever brand you like — just make sure it really works. True nonstick cookware should not require oils, sprays, or lard to stop items from sticking. This will benefit your waistline and your pH balance.

Reconsider what you're cooking your healthy, alkaline-forming meals in. Just as certain family heirloom skillets and glass decanters may contain lead, the American Cancer Society monitors research into whether an ingredient used in making a certain non-stick coating (can you say perfluorooctanoic acid three times fast) may release carcinogens when overheated. Alternatives include cookware labeled "non-toxic" or "green."

Clarifying your butter to stop suffocating your food

Heavy oils, butter, and cream don't accentuate the taste of healthy foods — they camouflage it. Get choosy about your oils — start a new trend. Sail past the shelves of lard, and head straight for the cold-pressed olive oil.

The words "cold pressed" will be small — you may need your readers if you're past 40 — but they will be somewhere on the label. Why cold pressed? Because it is the best of the olive oils — it wasn't heated, watered down, then reheated before going into that bottle you see on the shelf.

Although it is a good fatty acid, olive oil carries an extremely high calorie count. If you are watching your waistline, watch your olive oil consumption. Just one tablespoon can yield up to 200 calories, depending on the brand.

A word on butter: Even though it comes from milk, you can still use butter after you clarify it to remove the milk fats. You may know clarified butter as the drawn butter you get in a restaurant with your lobster or the delicious oily concoction on your popcorn.

To make it yourself, take a stick of unsalted butter and follow this recipe:

Clarified Butter

Prep time: 10 minutes • **Cook time:** 10 minutes • **Yield:** ¾ cup

Ingredients	Directions
3 sticks of unsalted butter	**1** Place the unsalted butter in a small, deep saucepan over low heat.
	2 After a few minutes, gently stir the melted butter. You should start to see a frothy concoction forming on the top — that's the milk fats.
	3 Using a tablespoon or small ladle, gently scoop the frothy milk fats and water off the top and discard. Continue to scoop and skim off the fats and water until only a pure, golden, clarified butter is left.
	4 Let the clarified butter cool for a few minutes, and then pour it into a glass container for storage.
	5 Store in the refrigerator. Make a big batch of clarified butter and store it in the fridge. You can use it just like regular butter or margarine (tablespoon for tablespoon). Aficionados swear it doesn't need to be refrigerated once the milk fats are removed, but I like my gastrointestinal system too much to take that chance.

Tip: Be sure to use a deep saucepan, otherwise you'll end up stirring the milk fats back in while you try to remove them. A deep pan allows you to skim them off the top easily.

Switching the grains

This transition is a difficult one, but once you get the hang of it, your pH will thank you. Wheat and whole wheat flour, white flour, rice — basically all refined starches — leave an acidic ash and wreck your pH. A hundred years ago, this may have been a major bummer. Today, you can find substitutes online, or if you're really savvy, you can find pH products pre-made for you in the health section.

My personal favorite exchange for white flour is a grain called *spelt*. Although you may not have heard of it, spelt is as old as the hills. It's similar to wheat, but with a nuttier flavor and less pH impact. You can find spelt in most health food stores and some of the larger grocery chains, in the form of ready-to-cook pastas and ground flour. If you don't have access to either of those, check online, where you can usually buy bigger quantities for less money.

The loaves of bread found in both supermarkets and convenience stores are chock-full of white or wheat flours, preservatives, and sugars — bad stuff. (I know, I know, I grew up on it, too). You have a few options when it comes to bread and pH. You can either use a pH friendly grain, such as spelt, to make your own, or you can look in the health food stores for breads that are yeast and wheat free. Personally, I like the Ezekiel brand — but you can choose whatever you like.

It's not just the grain that counts; it's the leavening agent wrecking your pH as well. Yeast is extremely acidifying.

If you want to use that homemade bread maker, seek out a recipe for unleavened bread and substitute your alkaline-friendly grains (spelt, barley, millet) for the white or whole wheat flour.

Sugar is a state of mind

This is the last painful exchange, I promise. But really, sugar is a state of mind. Some sweetener no-no's for your pH include:

- Artificial sweeteners (except Stevia)
- Brown sugar
- Powdered sugar
- Raw sugar

Let me introduce you to stevia, which is a natural sugar derived from the leaves of the sweet leaf plant (no, I didn't make that up). It's more potent that cane sugar, and little bits of it won't impact your pH. Stevia is available in most health food stores in powder and liquid form, depending on your preference (they both work great). If you just want to sweeten up a drink or smoothie, you can grow your own plant and use the dried, crumbled leaves. I hear that the plants are hardy and fairly difficult to kill!

Stevia doesn't have a one-to-one exchange ratio with sugar in recipes. If you're trying to substitute a stevia product for sugar, check the product's label for exchange advice. Too much stevia can ruin a recipe and impart a very bitter taste.

If you didn't know it was stevia and not sugar in that scrumptious cake, you wouldn't complain about it. Honestly, stevia tastes just as good, but isn't acidifying in your body in moderation.

Dehydrate this

If you don't have one, consider purchasing a dehydrator. A dehydrator helps you create shelves of healthy snacks such as kale chips, apple rings, banana chips — there aren't too many fruits or vegetables that cannot be successfully dehydrated for a great snack or pH-friendly condiment (think dried tomatoes on salad!).

Chapter 14

Breakfasts, Soups, and Salads

In This Chapter

▶ Whipping up breakfasts

▶ Sautéing splendid soups

▶ Sprucing up salads

When I started cooking, I needed a recipe to make hard-boiled eggs — ask my mother-in-law if you don't believe me. But these taste-tested, pH friendly meals that work perfectly for breakfast, lunch, or even a light dinner are user-friendly for even a kitchen klutz like me.

Feel free to exchange vegetables or proteins, but be careful to keep the exchanges alkaline-friendly (check Chapter 24 for some common swaps).

Whipping Up an Alkaline Breakfast

Breakfast is the most important meal of the day — fact, not a cliché. If you frequently skip breakfast, you may be adding unnecessary fluff to your waistline and stealing precious energy from your reserves.

A healthy breakfast should consist of a mixture of protein and carbohydrates (think a spinach and egg white omelet) to jump start your metabolism and fuel your brain for the day.

The next time you hit snooze and plan on skipping your first meal of the day, consider the consequences:

✔ Your energy and focus won't be up to par all day long.

✔ Your metabolism will stay slow, as if you were sleeping (breakfast jump-starts it).

✔ You will be tempted to over-indulge at lunch and supper, making up for lost calories.

✔ The vending machine will call to you.

✔ You may be more irritable, tired, and non-productive.

People who consistently skip breakfast usually have bigger waistlines and higher LDL (bad) cholesterol levels than those who start the day off right. And if you let your kids slide at breakfast-time, consider this: It's a proven fact that children who skip breakfast (30 percent of them don't eat it) have lower IQs in general and do not perform as well as the breakfast-eaters.

Whole eggs are a pH no-no on the acid alkaline diet. The yolks leave an acidic ash. If you have a hankering for a real hard-boiled egg, toss the yolk and eat only the white — problem solved.

Many of my breakfast recipes contain clarified butter, which takes only minutes to make and does not impact your pH like regular butter — check out Chapter 13 for the recipe.

Make sure you eat your breakfast within an hour of waking. After that, your body thinks you're starving and enters caveman mode. Your tissues begin to leech energy from your muscles, and your brain gets pretty unhappy as it's deprived of its main energy source — glucose, better known as sugar.

I'm hoping the breakfast recipes will tempt you to make your first meal of the day one of the tastiest, and deter you from skipping it.

Choices for breaking your fast

You ask, "Okay, I realize that I need to eat breakfast, but can it be something quick like cereal? How about one of those breakfast bars or shakes?" I answer, "Unfortunately, these temptingly convenient foods are probably not the best choice for your pH."

Although it may be better to eat something as opposed to nothing, healthy foods can be fast, as well. Chop up fruits and store them in bowls for a quick-grab in the morning. Cook your oats the night before (rolled oats take about 15 minutes).

Those choices are far less acidic than the hundreds of choices in the cereal aisle or the man-made powders and bars. Even most "healthy, whole-grain" cereals contain hoards of sugar, refined flours, and taste better paired with milk — a bowl of acidity waiting to happen.

Breakfast Scrambler

I love eggs with a capital "L," but they are an animal product, and therefore acidifying. In this recipe, I replace my beloved eggs with a block of firm tofu — it crumbles quite nicely and takes on the texture of soft scrambled eggs. Better yet, tofu is pretty hard to overcook, and it doesn't turn rubbery like eggs can.

Prep time: 15 minutes • **Cook time:** 20 minutes • **Yield:** 6-8 servings

Ingredients	*Directions*
2 tablespoons cold pressed olive oil, or clarified butter	*1* In a large nonstick skillet, cook the green and red peppers, asparagus, onion, garlic, and mushrooms in olive oil for 10 minutes, or until tender.
large green pepper, diced	
small red pepper, diced	*2* With your hands, crumble the block of tofu over the mixture and stir gently. Add the cumin, paprika, and crushed red pepper flakes and stir. Cover and cook for 10 more minutes, or until tofu is lightly browned.
3 stalks asparagus, finely chopped	
¼ cup diced cup yellow onion	
2 garlic cloves, pressed	*3* Add spinach leaves, stir, and cook until wilted.
1 cup sliced mushrooms	
16 ounce block of firm tofu, pressed	*4* Salt and pepper to taste.
¼ teaspoon cumin powder	
¼ teaspoon paprika	
¼ teaspoon crushed red pepper flakes	
½ cup raw spinach	
Salt and pepper to taste	

Per serving: Calories 103 (From Fat 65); Fat 7g (Saturated 1g); Cholesterol 0mg; Sodium 106mg; Carbohydrate 6g; Dietary Fiber 2g; Protein 6g.

Note: If you're not on the tofu train yet, don't worry. You can always exchange the block of tofu for six egg whites. Egg whites are less acidifying than the entire egg and lack the cholesterol and fat of the yolk.

Whey Good Smoothie

Oh and it is . . . way good. I love smoothies for three reasons. One, they are a convenient way to get a load of nutrients down quick. Two, you can drink them in your car on your way to work, school, or wherever the day takes you. Three, you can make them days ahead of time in the blender and store them in the fridge for daily use (but don't exceed three days; the enzymes in the fruits start to break down the smoothie and that's just gross).

Prep time: 5 minutes • **Yield:** 1 serving

Ingredients	Directions
1 cup soy or almond milk Handful of ice cubes 4 frozen strawberries, (if using fresh, add another handful of ice) 1 banana	**1** Put the milk, ice, strawberries, and banana in the blender and mix on medium (or coarse grind) until blended.
1-gram packet Stevia, or ¼ teaspoon powdered, or 6 drops of liquid, or ½ teaspoon fresh, minced leaves 1 scoop vanilla whey protein powder Few drops of vanilla extract	**2** Add stevia, protein powder, and the vanilla extract and pulse until blended. **3** Pour into a travel mug or cup and down your breakfast or yummy snack.

Per serving: Calories 324 (From Fat 56); Fat 6g (Saturated 2g); Cholesterol 26mg; Sodium 84mg; Carbohydrate 41g; Dietary Fiber 10g; Protein 30g.

Groovy Granola

Yes, I realize you can buy pre-made granola in the store . . . but it's not groovy, pH-lovin' granola. Store-bought granolas may contain added sugars, refined flours, preservatives, and other acidifying fillers.

You need to plan ahead — the almonds need to soak overnight before you can get started roasting. Make up a big batch for a great snack, smoothie topper, or a quick and nutritious breakfast.

Prep time: 10 minutes • **Cook time:** 20 minutes • **Yield:** 10 servings

Ingredients	Directions
3 cups raw almonds (soaked in water overnight)	**1** Strain almonds and blend in the food processor with the coconut and apricots.
½ cup shredded, unsweetened coconut	
½ cup dried apricots	**2** Place almond mixture in a large skillet saucepan over medium heat. Add rolled oats, stevia, and sea salt; stir.
2 cups rolled oats	
4 1-gram packets of Stevia, or 1 teaspoon powdered, or 1½ teaspoons fresh, minced leaves	**3** Roast over medium heat, stirring frequently, for about 15 minutes or until oats turn crisp.
Sprinkle of sea salt	**4** Spread the mixture out on parchment paper to cool. Store in an airtight container.

Per serving: Calories 368 (From Fat 234); Fat 26g (Saturated 4g); Cholesterol 0mg; Sodium 28mg; Carbohydrate 26g; Dietary Fiber 7g; Protein 13g.

Asparagus Omelet

Don't turn up your nose at asparagus. In this recipe, I'm not talking about the soaked-in-water-and-salt variety that you buy in the canned goods aisle; I'm talking about fresh, crisp asparagus spears paired with eggs.

This is one of the easiest, and most pH balanced omelets out there, thanks to the asparagus. Feel free to toss in some other alkalinizing vegetables; you would be surprised at how well your greens (think spinach, broccoli) complement egg whites in the morning.

Prep time: 5 minutes • **Cook time:** 10 minutes • **Yield:** 4 servings

Ingredients	*Directions*
6 egg whites (or egg substitute)	*1* In a small bowl, mix the egg whites, soy milk, and seasonings with a fork. Set aside.
2 tablespoons soy milk	
Dash black pepper	*2* In a large skillet, cook the asparagus in 1 tablespoon of the clarified butter over low-medium heat until tender (about 5 minutes). Remove the asparagus from the skillet and set it aside.
Dash garlic powder	
¼ teaspoon sea salt	
6 asparagus spears, diced	*3* Add the remaining 1 tablespoon of clarified butter to the skillet. Pour the egg mixture into the skillet and cook over low heat until it's slightly firm (about 5 minutes). Don't stir the mix — allow the eggs to set.
2 tablespoons clarified butter, divided	
	4 Using a spatula, gently lift and flip the omelet and cook the other side for another minute, or until the eggs are cooked through.
	5 Gently spoon cooked asparagus onto one half of the omelet and fold the other half over.

Per serving: Calories 89 (From Fat 59); Fat 7g (Saturated 4g); Cholesterol 16mg; Sodium 230mg; Carbohydrate 2g; Dietary Fiber 1g; Protein 6g.

Tip: If you have an oven-safe skillet, you can also bake your omelet (so it doesn't end up on the floor when you flip it). Bake at 350 degrees, uncovered, for about 35 minutes or until the eggs are set.

Bananas for Oatmeal

The men in my family can just dig into a bag of rolled oats and eat them like popcorn. Me — not so much. My taste buds require a little sweet and gooey to go with those dry oats.

Cook your rolled oats the night prior and you will be able to hit snooze one more time before making breakfast in the morning.

Prep time: 5 minutes • **Cook time:** 15 minutes • **Yield:** 2 servings

Ingredients	*Directions*
½ **cup soy or almond milk**	*1* In a medium saucepan, bring the milk, water, and oats to a boil.
½ **cup water**	
½ **cup rolled oats**	*2* Reduce heat to low and simmer for 5 to 10 minutes, or until oats are tender.
half a banana, mashed	
¼ **teaspoon cinnamon**	*3* Stir in the banana and cinnamon and cook for 1 minute longer.

Per serving: Calories 121 (From Fat 18); Fat 2g (Saturated .52g); Cholesterol 0mg; Sodium 39mg; Carbohydrate 23g; Dietary Fiber 3.5; Protein 4g.

Navigating egg substitutes

If you get that deer-in-the-headlight feeling while perusing the myriad fake egg selections, don't be discouraged. There are dozens of brands and flavors to choose from, but ultimately, your choice is a personal one. If your pH is staying in acid-land, it may be best to completely avoid real egg whites and stick to egg substitutes for a week or so. Consider your egg-tastic options:

✔ Commercial egg-free substitutes are a completely pH-safe alternative to real eggs, but I have to admit, the taste is not so great. Although you can find some of these products pre-made in the dairy section, the majority of egg replacements are found in health food stores or online, and come as a powder. Rather than using the water that most mixes call for, you can exchange soy or almond milk to add a little flavor to these mixes.

✔ Commercial egg-white products have far less impact on your pH than their shelled counterpart. Although these products are a bit pricey, it's quite nice to just pour out your egg whites as opposed to the messy process of separating them — and wasting all those yolks.

✔ Silken tofu has the consistency of yogurt and is a great egg-replacement in baked goods, or when you would use an egg for cohesiveness in a dish (think batter).

✔ Firm or crumbled tofu has the consistency of scrambled eggs and takes on the flavors of whatever it's cooked with. However, you can't make an omelet with firm tofu (that would be messy). If you're a visual eater, add a dash of turmeric to color your tofu "eggs" yellow.

Sautéing Splendid Soups

One of the best things about soup is that it usually fills you up before you can overindulge. If you need more than a bowl and spoon at your lunch or dinner table, trying pairing some of these recipes with a salad or some sprouted grain bread.

If you like to experiment (or have your own favorite soup recipe) keep these tips in mind:

- Any soup with the words "cream of" probably contains heavy creamers, sugars, and starches that are not pH friendly.

- Meat-based soups are okay every once in a while, if you stick to poultry or vegetable bases and avoid soups with a beef or red meat base.

- Get choosy about your vegetable broths — make sure the container says it's yeast-free. (Most organic vegetable broths are yeast free.)

- Use mashed vegetables or spelt flour as thickening agents.

Avoid arrowroot and cornstarch as thickening agents. Although they're convenient and easy to use (no lumps!), their starch component is acid-forming.

Making your own vegetable broth

Many alkalinizing recipes call for a vegetable broth base. If you don't want to use the canned, store-bought variety, consider making your own ahead of time. Vegetable bases are easy to make and can be stored in the refrigerator or freezer for future use.

Think about the flavors that get your mouth watering — is it the sweet onion, tangy tomato, or even the mellow staple of celery that calls to you? Most vegetable bases contain a combination of:

- Tomatoes
- Celery
- Onion

- Leek
- Carrot (go easy here, carrots can be acidifying)
- Cabbage
- Water
- Spices including salt, pepper, thyme, garlic, and bay leaves

Simmer your concoction on low for about 45 minutes, then let it cool. Strain the broth through cheesecloth to remove the chunks (who likes chunky broth?) and store in an airtight container.

Gazpacho

Gazpacho was a childhood favorite of mine. It wasn't until I started throwing together my own version of Mom's soup that I realized how little work was actually involved in making this refreshing chilled dish. I can remember snacking on bowls of the stuff after school; little did I know, Mom was serving up a healthy buffet of alkalinizing fruits and veggies. Let the soup sit in the fridge overnight to bring out the flavors.

Prep time: 15 minutes • **Cook time:** Let it chill overnight • **Yield:** 6 servings

Ingredients	*Directions*
1 small red onion, finely chopped	*1* Put the onions, tomatoes, and cucumbers in a food processor, and process until the vegetables are coarsely chopped.
46-ounce bottle tomato juice	
5 tomatoes	
1 cucumber, seeded	*2* Place processed mix in a large, non-metallic bowl, and add remaining ingredients; stir.
23 ounces Spicy V8 (½ of a 46-ounce bottle)	
1 small green bell pepper	*3* Place the soup in an airtight (non-metallic) container. Refrigerate overnight for maximum flavor.
2 cloves garlic, minced	
1 tablespoon fresh lemon juice	*4* Serve chilled with parsley garnish.
½ tablespoon sea salt	
Dash pepper	
Dash hot sauce (optional)	
1 tablespoon fresh parsley, finely chopped, or ½ tablespoon dried parsley	

Per serving: Calories 103 (From Fat 4); Fat 0g (Saturated 0g); Cholesterol 0mg; Sodium 1,484mg; Carbohydrate 21g; Dietary Fiber 3g; Protein 3g.

Tip: If you don't like things spicy, tone it down by omitting the Spicy V8 and hot sauce.

Fresh Veggie Soup

What could possibly be easier than simmering a bunch of fresh veggies and watching them merge into a delicious warm soup? Although it's crazy-simple, I included this recipe because I love the nutritional punch of vegetable soups, but had a hard time finding canned ones that didn't include a red meat base or fillers. If you are having a hard time finding "real" wild rice, check out the health food section.

Prep time: 10 minutes • **Cook time:** 30 minutes • **Yield:** 4 to 6 servings

Ingredients	Directions
1 tablespoon cold pressed olive oil	*1* In a small pan, sauté the onions in olive oil until translucent and set them aside.
1 small yellow onion, diced	
½ cup cooked wild rice	*2* Pour vegetable broth into large, heavy-bottomed pot and put over medium-low heat.
4 cups yeast-free vegetable broth	
1 zucchini, diced	*3* Add the remaining ingredients, including the rice and onions, and simmer, uncovered, for 30 minutes.
1 stalk celery	
4 plum tomatoes, seeded and diced	*4* Remove the celery stalk and peppercorns by skimming them off the top of the soup with a small-slotted spoon and discard them.
½ cup frozen, chopped spinach	
Dash of sea salt to taste	*5* Garnish with fresh parsley, if desired, and pair with sprouted grain tortillas.
5 whole peppercorns	
Fresh parsley (optional)	

Per serving: Calories 91 (From Fat 39); Fat 4g (Saturated 1g); Cholesterol 0mg; Sodium 679mg; Carbohydrate 12g; Dietary Fiber 3g; Protein 4g.

Hearty Chicken Soup

I hesitated in listing this filling recipe, knowing I am sure to upset at least a handful of steadfast pH dieters by telling you to add meat to a recipe. You *can* eat animal proteins — you just have to do so in very limited moderation (remember the 80/20 rule that I talk about in Chapter 2). This hearty soup will feed a family of six, and it calls for only two chicken breasts; it's pH- and wallet-friendly.

Prep time: 15 minutes • **Cook time:** 45 minutes • **Yield:** 6 servings

Ingredients	*Directions*
½ **cup wild rice**	*1* Cook the wild rice according to package directions and set it aside.
1 yellow onion, finely chopped	
2 cloves garlic, pressed	*2* In a small pan, cook the onions and garlic in clarified butter over low heat until the onion is translucent.
2 tablespoons clarified butter	
2 cooked chicken breasts, diced	*3* In a large pot, cook the chicken, vegetable stock, water, celery, and seasonings on medium-low. Add the sautéed garlic and onions and the wild rice. Simmer for 20 minutes.
4 cups yeast-free vegetable stock	
2 cups water	
1 celery stalk, finely chopped	*4* Add the endive and cook another 5 minutes, or until the endive is wilted.
½ **tablespoon thyme**	
½ **teaspoon sea salt**	*5* Stir in the spelt flour and bring to a low boil for 2 minutes, constantly stirring.
3 bay leaves	
Dash pepper	*6* Remove and discard the bay leaves and serve your soup!
½ **cup chopped endive**	
2 tablespoons spelt flour	

Per serving: Calories 138 (From Fat 18); Fat 2g (Saturated 0g); Cholesterol 24mg; Sodium 891mg; Carbohydrate 19g; Dietary Fiber 2g; Protein 13g.

Lean, Mean Chili Machine

This dish comes to your table at the expense of my family's taste buds. When I dropped meat from my diet, I spent many a night ordering takeout while my husband kindly dumped the awful, vegetarian chili I'd fixed down the disposal. These horrific concoctions looked so good in the cans or powdered mixes at the grocery store, but failed miserably on the dinner table. Our taste buds were finally assuaged one evening, when the planets aligned and I got my mixture right. You're welcome.

If you're using raw lentils, you need to soak them. Traditionally, you do this in water overnight, but for a fast soak, you can place the lentils in a large pot and cover them with water. Bring the water to a boil, then turn off the water and let the lentils sit for about two hours.

Prep time: 10 minutes • **Cook time:** 15 minutes • **Yield:** 4 servings

Ingredients	*Directions*
32 oz. lentils, raw or drained canned	*1* Cook raw lentils according to package directions, set aside. *(Or use canned.)*
28-ounce can diced tomatoes, drained, or 3 cups diced fresh	*2* In a small pan, sauté onions, green and red peppers, and garlic in clarified butter until onions are translucent.
1 small red onion, chopped	
1 green bell pepper, chopped	
1 red bell pepper, chopped	*3* Put the onions and pepper mix in a large heavy-bottomed pot, then add lentils and all of the remaining ingredients except for the cheese and bring the soup to a boil.
2 garlic cloves, minced	
1 tablespoon clarified butter	
½ cup salsa	*4* Simmer for 15 minutes on low, or until vegetables are tender but firm.
1 cup tomato juice	
1 cup water	*5* Top with fat-free cheddar cheese, if you like.
3 tablespoons chili powder	
¼ teaspoon cayenne pepper	
½ teaspoon black pepper	
½ teaspoon sea salt	
Dash stevia powder, or 2 drops liquid, or 1 minced, fresh leaf	
¼ cup fat-free cheddar cheese (optional)	

Per serving: Calories 908 (From Fat 68); Fat 7g (Saturated 3g); Cholesterol 8mg; Sodium 1,029mg; Carbohydrate 154g; Dietary Fiber 76g; Protein 68g.

Tip: Hollow out small pie pumpkins and use them as chili bowls for a fun autumn treat.

Meatless Minestrone

I'm not Italian, but I make a mean minestrone. The problem is, most traditional recipes call for ground beef or chuck, which you want to avoid (even in small amounts). My secret? Capture the *umami,* which is the meat-like essence, using a few key ingredients. After a few bites, your family won't even notice that they are eating meatless minestrone.

Prep time: 15 minutes • **Cook time:** 30 minutes • **Yield:** 4 to 6 servings

Ingredients	Directions
½ cup chopped yellow onion	**1** In a large pot, cook the onions, bell pepper, garlic, and carrot in 2 tablespoons of clarified butter until onions are transparent.
1 green bell pepper, diced	
4 garlic cloves, pressed	
1 small carrot, grated	**2** Stir in the remaining vegetables — the cabbage, tomatoes, and zucchini — and tomato sauce. Sauté everything for 3 to 5 minutes, or until the cabbage starts to wilt. Add the remaining 2 tablespoons of clarified butter if the mixture is dry or sticking to the pan.
4 tablespoons clarified butter, divided	
1 cup cabbage, chopped	
14.5-ounce can of diced tomatoes	**3** Slowly pour in the vegetable stock and water, add the bay leaf, basil, soy sauce, and uncooked shell pasta. Mix thoroughly but gently and bring to a boil.
1 small zucchini, diced	
12 oz. tomato sauce	
2 cups yeast-free vegetable stock	**4** Cook at a low boil for 5 to 7 minutes, or until pasta is tender.
1 cup water	
1 teaspoon fresh basil, chopped	**5** Garnish with parmesan cheese, if desired.
½ teaspoon soy sauce	
1 bay leaf	
1 cup uncooked spelt pasta shells	
1 tablespoon parmesan cheese	

Per serving: Calories 198 (From Fat 67); Fat 8g (Saturated 4g); Cholesterol 16mg; Sodium 1,098mg; Carbohydrate 30g; Dietary Fiber 7g; Protein 7g.

Spicing Up Your Salads: A pH Staple

If you're the kind of person who thinks "iceberg and ranch" when someone says "salad," prepare for a new reality. Unless you throw grilled steak on top, there aren't many mistakes you can make, pH-wise, with this basic staple. Salads are a great way add fruits and veggies to any meal and can be very visually pleasing.

The first step in becoming a salad connoisseur is getting to know your green leafies. The darker the leaf, the more nutrients it has. So, as this guide tells you, iceberg has very little in the way of vitamins and minerals. The green leafy plants at the cornerstone of any good, garden salad include:

- ✔ Arugula
- ✔ Butter, also known as Boston lettuce
- ✔ Endive
- ✔ Iceberg lettuce
- ✔ Kale (eat raw only if you are a guinea pig; kale is bitter!)
- ✔ Oak leaf lettuce
- ✔ Romaine lettuce, regular or hearts
- ✔ Spinach, regular or baby
- ✔ Watercress

Simple soups

Back in my grandmother's day, soups were a way of saving the budget while feeding a large family. Ingredients were not choice — they were a hodgepodge of leftovers from the nights prior. Chicken bones would feed the family for days, paired with a couple cups of water and simmered for hours.

Nothing has changed; you can still feed a large family on a tight budget using soup. I don't have a culinary degree to make tasty soups, and you don't need one either. Choose from any of the following ingredients, simmer them for at least 30 minutes and voila! You have soup.

- ✔ **Greens:** Spinach, kale, cabbage, broccoli, green beans, celery, leeks, endive, asparagus
- ✔ **Perfect proteins:** Vegetable stock, silken tofu, chicken stock (sparingly), egg whites, lentils
- ✔ **Fillers:** Small diced potatoes (sparingly), wild rice, spelt pasta, onions, zucchini, tomatoes, garlic

The list of combinations is virtually endless, as long as you avoid acidifying vegetables such as corn.

Spinach Medley

The word _medley_ means an assortment, a mix. That's exactly what this spinach medley salad is — a harmonious mix of ingredients that don't sound complementary (but they are). Raw spinach leaves are my favorite salad base. They contain a mix of delicious phytochemicals and nutrients that produce that vibrant green coloring. Although we grow ours in an outside patio pot (it's as easy as growing grass), you can buy bags of pre-washed spinach at the grocery store. Vibrant green leaves, warm brown roasted pine nuts, hidden herbs and a splash of orange tangerines make this salad pleasing to your peepers as well as your taste buds.

Prep time: 15 minutes • **Cook time:** 10 minutes • **Yield:** 4 servings

Ingredients	Directions
3 cups raw spinach leaves	_1_ In a large salad bowl, mix the spinach, endive, basil, parsley, and onion slices. Set aside.
1 cup endive	
1 tablespoon fresh chopped basil	_2_ In a small sauté pan, melt the clarified butter over low heat. Add the shrimp and lime and warm them for 1 minute. (Don't overcook shrimp — they get chewy.)
1 tablespoon fresh chopped parsley	
¼ small red onion, sliced in rings	_3_ Top the salad bowl mix with the shrimp, pine nuts, and dressing of your choice, then toss to mix.
1 tablespoon clarified butter	
½ cup ready-to-eat medium-sized shrimp (tails removed)	_4_ Garnish the salad with the tangerine wedges and serve.
2 small tangerines, peeled and sectioned	
¼ cup roasted pine nuts (see the following roasting directions)	
1 teaspoon fresh lime juice	

**Per serving:** Calories 239 (From Fat 193); Fat 22g (Saturated 5g); Cholesterol 35mg; Sodium 48mg; Carbohydrate 7g; Dietary Fiber 2g; Protein 7g.

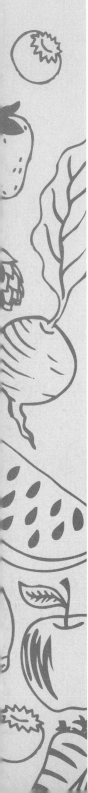

Roasted Pine Nuts

¼ cup pine nuts

1 teaspoon cold pressed olive oil

1 Toss the pine nuts in olive oil.

2 Heat a medium skillet over medium-low heat and add the pine nuts.

3 Roast for 5 to 10 minutes, or until lightly browned.

Spinach Salad Dressing

¼ cup lemon juice

¼ teaspoon fresh ground pepper

1 clove garlic, pressed

¼ cup cold pressed olive oil

¼ teaspoon fresh chopped basil, or ⅛ teaspoon dried basil

1 teaspoon fresh chopped parsley, or ½ teaspoon dried parsley

½ of 1-gram packet Stevia, or ⅛ teaspoon powder, or 3 drops liquid, or 1 fresh, minced leaf (optional)

1 Combine all the ingredients in a small bowl and mix thoroughly.

Getting rings from fresh pineapple

I love pineapples but don't want the ones that taste of aluminum (canned). In Hawaii, I learned the proper procedure to get pineapple rings from a fresh pineapple. It's not challenging, once you know what you're doing! Just follow these steps:

1. Purchase fresh pineapples at the grocer. Smell the fruit (looks weird but it works). If it smells sweet but doesn't have gnats hovering, you've got a good, ripe pineapple.

2. At home, grab the pineapple in one hand and the stem in the other and give a firm twist. The stem will pop off.

3. Peel the pineapple with a sharp, serrated knife. Remove any remaining hard spots or spikes with a smaller paring knife.

4. If you have a pineapple corer, use it to remove the tough core of the pineapple. If you do not, slice the pineapple into rings, then remove the tough center core with a paring knife.

Sweet 'N' Sour Salad

Your tongue is covered in thousands of specialized taste buds. Thanks to your tongue, nose, and saliva, your brain can process sweet, salty, and sour foods all at once. Fire up the grill to enjoy this salad that includes grilled pineapple and pecans wrapped in ginger on a bed of greens.

Prep time: 20 minutes • **Cook time:** 10 minutes • **Yield:** 4 servings

Ingredients	*Directions*
1 cup spinach **1 cup butter lettuce** **6 pineapple rings (fresh or canned)**	*1* Spray the highest rack in the grill with non-stick cooking spray (before turning it on). Heat the grill to medium-low. Lay pineapple slices on the grill and cook for 3 minutes per side. Set aside.
½ cup watercress **1 green bell pepper, sliced in rings**	*2* Rip or cut greens into bite-sized pieces. In a large salad bowl, mix spinach, butter lettuce, and watercress.
½ cup gingered pecans (see following recipe)	*3* Top salad with green bell pepper rings, grilled pineapple, and gingered pecans. Add a splash of cold-pressed olive oil, if desired, for added moisture.

Per serving: Calories 214 (From Fat 155); Fat 17g (Saturated 2g); Cholesterol 0mg; Sodium 302mg; Carbohydrate 16g; Dietary Fiber 4g; Protein 3g.

Gingered Pecans

1-gram packet Stevia, or ¼ teaspoon powdered, or 6 drops of liquid, or ½ teaspoon fresh, minced leaves	*1* Mix the stevia, sea salt, and ginger in small bowl. Set aside.
½ teaspoon sea salt **¼ teaspoon ginger powder** **4 tablespoons water**	*2* In a small pan, bring the water and olive oil to a slow boil over medium heat. Add the pecans and stevia mixture to the pan and continue to boil until the liquid is evaporated, stirring constantly.
½ tablespoon cold pressed olive oil **½ cup pecan halves**	*3* Pour the pecans onto paper towels and let dry.

Antipasto

Any time you resist the urge to cook your veggies and eat them in their raw state, you are ingesting even higher amounts of phytochemicals than in the cooked version — this is a good thing. When you cook your veggies, some of the phytochemicals are killed with the heat — making your naturally nutritious food *less* nutritious!

Phytochemicals are the lovely chemicals that protect plant foods from disease and give them their pretty bright colors. They keep popping up in science, as we try to isolate which phytochemicals help fight what — and put them in a pill.

Prep time: 15 minutes • **Cook time:** 10 minutes • **Yield:** 4 servings

Ingredients	Directions
1 cup cooked spelt pasta	*1* Toss the cooled pasta with the other ingredients, except the dressing, in a large bowl.
½ green bell pepper, diced	
½ red bell pepper, diced	
½ pound of lentils, fresh, cooked or canned and drained	*2* Pour the Antipasto Dressing over the pasta mixture and toss to coat. Place the salad in an airtight container in the refrigerator for 2 to 4 hours.
1 small firm avocado, diced	
1 small red onion, coarsely chopped	*3* Check the antipasto after 2 hours. If it seems dry, add an additional ½ cup olive oil and toss to coat, then return to fridge overnight.
½ cup broccoli, trimmed into bite-size chunks	
Antipasto Dressing (see recipe following the Broccoli Salad recipe)	

Per serving: Calories 574 (From Fat 321); Fat 36g (Saturated 5g); Cholesterol 0mg; Sodium 300mg; Carbohydrate 51g; Dietary Fiber 18g; Protein 19g.

Tip: Resist the temptation to add the traditional olives or salami; they'll turn this dish from alkalinizing to acidifying.

Broccoli Salad

You've probably seen broccoli salad with the bacon and creamy mayonnaise-based sauce disappear pretty quickly at parties. Unfortunately, that crowd-pleaser is pretty tough on your acid base balance. This is a pH-friendly dish, and you can serve it with or without the blender-friendly, Almond-aise mayo-substitute, depending on how much time you want to spend in the kitchen.

Prep time: 20 minutes • **Cook time:** 5 minutes • **Yield:** 4 servings

Ingredients	Directions
3 slices turkey bacon (optional, but good)	*1* Cook turkey bacon per package directions, preferably until crisp. Lay on paper towels to dry.
2 cups broccoli cut into bite-sized florets	*2* Mix the broccoli, cauliflower, tomatoes, and almonds in large bowl, toss with ½ cup of the Almond-aise. Refrigerate for at least 6 hours, preferably overnight.
½ cup cauliflower florets	
½ cup halved cherry tomatoes	
½ cup sliced almonds	*3* Serve chilled, garnished with crumbled bacon and the green pepper rings.
½ green bell pepper, sliced in rings	
Almond-aise (see following recipe)	

Per serving: Calories 407 (From Fat 352); Fat 39g (Saturated 5g); Cholesterol 0mg; Sodium 63mg; Carbohydrate 12g; Dietary Fiber 6g; Protein 8g.

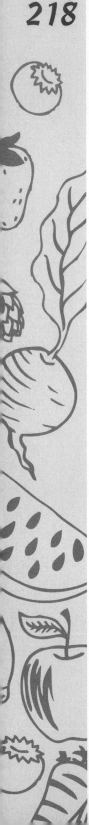

Almond-aise

¼ cup apple cider vinegar

5 tablespoons water

Dash sea salt

½ teaspoon garlic powder

30 almonds

½ cup cold-pressed olive oil

1 Place the apple cider vinegar, water, salt, and garlic in a blender and mix on low for 1 minute.

2 Slowly add the almonds, five at a time and pulse on high to crush.

3 Drizzle in the olive oil and blend on low, until the mixture becomes creamy and mayonnaise-like.

Antipasto Dressing

½ cup cold-pressed olive oil

¼ cup lemon juice

2 cloves of garlic, pressed

½ teaspoon sea salt

¼ teaspoon pepper

1 teaspoon fresh chopped basil, or ½ teaspoon dried

½ teaspoon fresh oregano, or ¼ teaspoon dried

1-gram packet Stevia, or ¼ teaspoon powder, or 6 drops liquid, or ½ teaspoon fresh, minced leaves

1 In a shaker bottle or a small bowl, mix all the ingredients thoroughly.

Fabulous Fruit Salad

After just a few bites, I bet you never turn to that syrupy canned concoction again. This recipe calls for some easy-to-find fresh fruits, although they may vary by season (apricots). Feel free to substitute your own favorites, staying away from (or using sparingly) acidifying fruits such as cherries, plums, and cranberries.

Prep time: 15 minutes • **Yield:** 4 to 6 servings

Ingredients	Directions
2 1-gram packets Stevia, or ½ teaspoon powder, or 10 drops liquid, or 1 teaspoon fresh, minced leaves	**1** In a small bowl, mix the stevia, lemon juice, and yogurt. Set aside.
2 teaspoons lemon juice	
1 cup nonfat soy yogurt	**2** In a large bowl, toss the fruits and top them with the yogurt mixture. Place in the refrigerator to chill for 2 hours.
1 cantaloupe, cut into bite-sized wedges	
1 cup bite-size pieces of honeydew melon	**3** Serve chilled, garnished with the slivered almonds.
½ cup pineapple chunks	
4 apricots, pitted and quartered	
2 small oranges, in wedges	
¼ cup slivered almonds	

Per serving: Calories 226 (From Fat 43); Fat 5g (Saturated 0g); Cholesterol 0mg; Sodium 77mg; Carbohydrate 42g; Dietary Fiber 4g; Protein 6g.

Making spreads simple

True or false: On the acid alkaline diet, your sandwiches will be boring, and you cannot eat spreads. False! You can easily experiment with making your own spreads. All you need is a blender and an imagination. Try making different spreads for fruit salads, vegetables, and sandwiches using a combination of:

- Almond or soy milk
- Almonds or almond flour
- Apple cider vinegar
- Cold-pressed olive oil
- Cucumbers
- Lemon juice
- Nonfat soy yogurt
- Spices and herbs including sea salt, pepper, garlic powder, curry, and dill
- Tofutti "Better Than Cream Cheese"

A word of caution about store-bought "egg-free" or "gluten-free" mayonnaise: Many of them have a canola oil base and use acidifying fillers, such as white flour or other starches. And be aware that purchasing the product in a health food store does not guarantee that it's good for your pH. You will never go wrong if you stop and read the label.

Chapter 15

Munching on Mains: Filling Up on the Right Stuff

*Y*ou may be thinking it's much easier to whip up a box of noodle-os and ground meat for dinner — or is it? I am not a chef. I am a working mother with a family to feed, and I do have a social life. I don't spend all my time in the kitchen, and you won't have to either. If you know the upcoming week is going to be crazy, consider taking a page from my mother-in-law's book, and spend Sunday baking and freezing entrees for the week.

Whatever you choose for dinner tonight, you can manipulate almost any recipe into an acid alkaline one with a little finesse. It's all about healthy exchanges and putting more alkalinizing foods on the plate.

Preparing the "Other" White Non-Meat

I am not sure what the tofu discrimination is all about. There are many reasons to adore it.

✔ It's versatile and takes on the flavor of the dish.

✔ You can use it crumbled or in slices, like meat.

✔ It has very low calories per serving.

- ✔ Tofu has zero cholesterol or animal fat.

- ✔ It is a good source of calcium and protein.

- ✔ You won't get sick from touching it raw.

Many of my friends literally gag when I tell them how much I love this vegetable protein (I even had one threaten not to visit if I made her eat it), but I
love it just the same.

Tofu is a vegetable protein derived from soybeans. Unlike some beloved
meat, it does not contain ground up tongue or anything weird — just soybean
curds. Some savvy grocers and most health food stores have shelves of the
stuff in many different preparations including:

- ✔ **Silken tofu,** which has a yogurt-like consistency and works great in
  smoothies and baked dishes, especially if that dish requires a little extra
  protein.

- ✔ **Firm** and **extra firm tofu** comes in a small block shape and can be sliced
  to mimic pieces of meat for grilling, frying, sautéing, or even baking.

- ✔ **Tofu crumbles** are a variation of medium-firm tofu crumbled into a
  scrambled-egg-like consistency. They work great in stir-frys and baked
  dishes.

- ✔ **Fake meats** including versions of hot dogs, sausages, and chicken patties
  are usually a blend of tofu, lentils, and vegetables.

Firm tofu comes in a vacuum-sealed pack filled with water. To get a block
ready for cooking:

1. **Open the pack and drain the water.**

2. **Rinse the tofu block in running water.**

3. **Wrap a clean kitchen towel around the block.**

4. **Press the wrapped tofu between two clean plates to drain excess
   water so that the tofu is a little drier and more meat-like.**

Put unused tofu in a small container, cover it completely with water, and
store it in the refrigerator. Change the water daily (otherwise it stinks and
gets cloudy) and the remaining tofu will last about a week.

You can freeze blocks of tofu. It will darken in color and toughen a little — but
it is still perfectly okay to eat, and some people like the texture better after it's
been frozen.

Stuffed Green Peppers

Whether you cook them quickly in the oven or let them stew all day in a crock pot, nothing compares to the homey aroma of stuffed green peppers at your dinner table. I've included the oven recipe here, but the slow cooker recipe is similar (do not pre-cook the green peppers, cook on medium-low for 6 hours). Green peppers are a natural source of vitamin C, and they're great alkalinizers. If you have trouble finding basmati rice, you can substitute wild rice, rolled oats, bulgur, or quinoa.

Prep time: 20 minutes • **Cook time:** 40 minutes • **Yield:** 6 servings

Ingredients	*Directions*
6 green bell peppers	*1* Preheat the oven to 350 degrees.
10 cups water	
1 pound tofu crumbles	*2* Wash the peppers then cut the top off of each. Using a small paring knife, remove the stems from the pepper tops and dice the tops finely. Set the diced peppers aside. Remove the seeds and light membranes from the intact peppers.
1 clove garlic, pressed	
¼ white onion, chopped	
¼ teaspoon sea salt	
¼ teaspoon black pepper	*3* Pour the water into a large pot. Submerge the peppers in the water, making sure that the peppers sit up, so the water floods into them. Bring the peppers to a low boil and boil for 7 minutes. Drain the peppers and set them aside to cool.
Splash of soy sauce	
½ teaspoon chili powder	
1 cup cooked basmati rice	*4* Preheat a large nonstick skillet to medium. Add the tofu crumbles, garlic, diced green pepper tops, white onion, salt, and pepper, and cook for 5 minutes, stirring frequently.
2 cans stewed tomatoes	
¼ cup nonfat mozzarella cheese (optional)	*5* Add a splash of soy sauce (or to taste), the chili pepper, basmati rice, and one can of stewed tomatoes to the skillet. Simmer on low for 5 minutes.
	6 Arrange the cooked peppers standing up in a large baking dish. Spoon the tofu and rice mixture into each pepper, gently pressing down with the back of the spoon to stuff each one to the top.
	7 Pour the remaining can of stewed tomatoes on and around the peppers. Sprinkle them with mozzarella cheese and bake for 20 minutes or until cheese starts to brown.

Per serving: Calories 160 (From Fat 28); Fat 3g (Saturated 0g); Cholesterol 0mg; Sodium 549mg; Carbohydrate 30g; Dietary Fiber 5g; Protein 8g.

Tip: Basmati rice is cooked similar to wild rice, taking about 15 to 20 minutes. Prepare a batch ahead of time and store it covered in the refrigerator for less preparation and cooking time.

Veggie Bake

Nothing says working parent like a casserole, but this one isn't boring. You can prepare it days ahead of time and toss it in the oven when hunger pangs for a healthy meal kick in. I love this kind of standalone meal that doesn't dump a million dirty dishes in the sink. And by the way, no one will know you're feeding them tofu unless you want to tell.

Prep time: 15 minutes • **Cook time:** 60 minutes • **Yield:** 6 servings

Ingredients	Directions
1 tablespoon cold-pressed olive oil	*1* Preheat the oven to 350 degrees. Grease a large 9-x-13 baking dish with the olive oil.
1 block firm tofu, pressed	
3 egg whites	*2* In a large bowl, mash the block of tofu with a potato masher.
2 cups broccoli florets	
2 garlic cloves, pressed	*3* Pour in the egg whites and stir well.
¼ cup diced yellow onion	
1 cup raw spinach	*4* Add the remaining ingredients and mix everything together. Spoon the mixture into the greased baking dish and bake, uncovered, for 1 hour.
10 mushrooms, sliced	
1 teaspoon crushed red pepper	
½ teaspoon powdered ginger	
1 teaspoon soy sauce	
1 cup raw spinach	

Per serving: Calories 92 (From Fat 45); Fat 5g (Saturated 1g); Cholesterol 0mg; Sodium 43mg; Carbohydrate 6g; Dietary Fiber 2g; Protein 8g.

Introducing Veggie-Based Dinners

No longer are vegetables relegated to side dishes or integrated as afterthoughts. In the acid alkaline diet, vegetables take center stage and are frequently the main entrée. You can never go wrong adding more of these plant foods to your plate, or snacking on them throughout the day when hunger strikes. Watch out — you may become a full-fledged vegetarian while transitioning to a pH friendly diet. After all, the diets are very similar.

The only trick I use while cooking is my knowledge of how to pair good proteins, such as three ounces of chicken breast, tofu, or salmon, with tons of vegetables (but I may still be a magician, because my kids do love to eat these veggies).

Does it end in -ase?

Raw plant foods contain a heap of healthy enzymes — think of them as microscopic firecrackers that spark chemical reactions throughout your body. Although they are not a dietary staple (your body makes human enzymes), healthy plant enzymes boost your immune function and digestive process. Want to know how to spot an enzyme? Almost all of them end with the suffix –ase. Don't believe me? During digestion:

✔ Amyl**ase** breaks down sugars

✔ Prote**ase** breaks down protein

✔ Cellul**ase** breaks down carbs

✔ Lip**ase** breaks down fat

Ever overcook a green bell pepper? It turns a foul green color — you killed the enzymes. Just like us, enzymes are delicate creatures who need the right temperature, pH, and water to survive. To retain more of these helpful enzymes in your plant foods:

✔ Eat them raw.

✔ Chew your food thoroughly (stimulates more amylase for good digestion).

✔ Steam your veggies.

✔ If you're boiling vegetables, do it briefly — a 3-minute blanche instead of a 10-minute rolling boil.

✔ Stir fry vegetables.

✔ Puree raw fruits and veggies and have a smoothie.

And if you want to feast on enzymes, try some sprouted foods. Any grain, lentil, or seed has its peak enzyme content while it is sprouting including:

✔ Alfalfa

✔ Flax

✔ Broccoli (go figure)

✔ Mung beans

Add them to a salad, sandwich, wrap, or smoothie to get a boost of healthy plant enzymes.

Zucchini Quesadillas

Quesadillas are like the grilled cheese of this century. They are fast, filling, and really hard to screw up. The secret is to locate the right tortillas for your pH — not any old flour, corn, or wheat-based one will do. Check out the health food section or go online. You want to make sure the tortillas are sprouted, whole grain, *and* flour-less.

Prep time: 10 minutes • **Cook time:** 15 minutes • **Yield:** 4 to 6 servings

Ingredients	Directions
¼ cup clarified butter or cold-pressed olive oil, divided 4 cups diced zucchini 1 cup chopped yellow onion 1 teaspoon fresh chopped parsley 1 teaspoon crushed red pepper 1 teaspoon garlic powder Sprinkle sea salt Dash hot sauce 8 8-inch sprouted grain tortillas ½ cup fat-free mozzarella (or soy cheese)	**1** Heat a tablespoon of clarified butter in a large skillet over medium heat. Add the diced zucchini and onions. Cook until tender. **2** Remove the skillet from the heat and stir in the parsley, red pepper, garlic powder, sea salt, and hot sauce. Return the skillet to the stove and warm the veggie-spice mixture on low for 1 to 2 minutes until it's heated through. **3** Grease another large skillet with a quarter of the remaining clarified butter. Heat the skillet over medium-low and place a tortilla in the pan. Spoon the zucchini mixture evenly over the tortilla and sprinkle it with cheese. Top with another tortilla. **4** Use a spatula to gently lift one edge of the bottom tortilla and flip it when the center is browned and slightly crispy. Cook the other side until the bottom is browned and crisp. **5** Remove the quesadilla from pan, and use a pizza cutter to cut it into wedges. **6** Repeat Steps 3 though 5 with the remaining zucchini mix and tortillas. Serve with fresh salsa, if desired.

Per serving: Calories 472 (From Fat 127); Fat 14g (Saturated 8g); Cholesterol 35mg; Sodium 564mg; Carbohydrate 63g; Dietary Fiber 13g; Protein 24g.

Making Pizza Pie: A Two-Part Process

If there were no pizza on the acid alkaline diet, I would not be on it. Pizza should be considered a dietary staple — a comfort food — that you can indulge in weekly. But when you're on the acid alkaline diet, not any old pizza will do, and most certainly not the ones in the freezer section that are brimming over with yeast, white flour, preservatives, fatty cheeses, and who knows what else.

Digging into dough

The carb-a-holic in you may be hesitant to start this diet if I told you that your dough days were over. Actually, that's only half true. You do need to forgo yeasty, refined dough, but a nice thin-crust pizza is just the ticket. This dough recipe started out as a recipe for focaccia bread, but then I said what the heck, this might make a delicious pizza. Boy, was I right!

Stirring up the sauce

Pizza sauce is an easy gourmet treat. You can top a sheet of doughy deliciousness with olive oil and spices, tomatoes, and cheeses — whatever gets you happy. Just for the fun of it, I'm throwing in an alkaline pizza sauce recipe. It will take a whole 2 minutes to throw together and is missing the preservatives and sodium found in most commercial brands.

Hold the Acids Pizza Dough

Prep time: 15 minutes • **Cook time:** 25 minutes • **Yield:** 8 servings

Ingredients	*Directions*
3 tablespoons cold-pressed olive oil, divided	*1* Preheat the oven to 425 degrees. Grease a 9-x-13 baking sheet with 1 tablespoon of olive oil.
2 cups spelt flour	
2 teaspoons baking powder	*2* In a medium-sized bowl, combine spelt flour, baking powder, sea salt, garlic powder, rosemary, and parmesan. Set aside.
½ teaspoon sea salt	
½ teaspoon garlic powder	
1 teaspoon dried rosemary, or 2 teaspoons fresh, minced	*3* In a small bowl, combine the water and ½ teaspoon of olive oil; stir this mixture into the center of the dry mix, then knead the dough with oiled hands until it becomes sticky.
1 tablespoon parmesan cheese	
1 cup room temperature water	*4* Spread the dough onto the greased baking sheet in a uniform thickness. Dimple the dough surface every 1 to 2 inches using your thumb. Rub remaining olive oil over the surface and bake for 25 minutes.

Per serving: Calories 134 (From Fat 37); Fat 4g (Saturated 1g); Cholesterol 1mg; Sodium 470mg; Carbohydrate 24g; Dietary Fiber 5g; Protein 4g.

Note: You don't have to pre-bake the crust prior to topping it, but I find that the pre-bake stops soggy dough. Nobody wants to eat a soggy pizza pie!

Pass the Pizza Sauce

Prep time: 5 minutes • **Yield:** 1 pizza

Ingredients	Directions
14½-ounce can diced tomatoes, drained 3 cloves garlic, pressed 1 teaspoon fresh chopped parsley, or ½ teaspoon dried 1 teaspoon crushed red pepper 6-ounce can tomato paste 1 teaspoon garlic powder Sprinkle sea salt Dash hot sauce	*1* In a medium bowl, mix together all ingredients and let stand for at least 15 minutes before spreading it on a Hold the Acids Pizza Dough crust (see the preceding recipe).

Per serving: Calories 19 (From Fat 1); Fat 0g (Saturated 0g); Cholesterol 0mg; Sodium 108mg; Carbohydrate 4g; Dietary Fiber 1g; Protein 1g. (Based on 8 servings.)

Tip: The longer you let the sauce sit, the better it tastes. But put it in the fridge if you are going to let it rest longer than 15 minutes.

Sprucing up your pie with roasted garlic

For a naked pizza (no sauce, just brushed olive oil), consider garnishing your dough with fresh chunks of tomato or cloves of freshly roasted garlic.

If you don't know how to roast a clove of garlic, you may be missing out on a healthy treat! This plant is bursting with antioxidants and is under constant scientific scrutiny for its role in fighting disease. Aside from staving off hungry vampires, garlic is being studied for its myriad benefits that may include:

✔ Reducing cardiovascular disease

✔ Improving immune function

✔ Decreasing high cholesterol

✔ Fighting the common cold

When a bulb of garlic is roasted, the cloves slip right out of the skin and have the consistency of butter at room temperature. You can leave them whole or mash them into a paste to flavor your foods. Just be sure to have some breath mints on hand! To roast a bulb of garlic:

1. Slice off the very bottom of the garlic bulb, exposing the cloves. Do not peel the bulb.

2. Place one tablespoon of cold-pressed olive oil in a small, oven-safe dish.

3. Sprinkle sea salt and pepper in the olive oil if desired and place the garlic, cut side down, in the dish.

4. Roast at 350 degrees for 30 to 45 minutes, or until desired consistency achieved. (The longer you roast, the gooier the garlic cloves become.)

Veggie Pizza Pie

Just like the sun will rise tomorrow, a real pizza must have cheese. Lucky for you, this recipe effortlessly balances the acidifying cheese, which comprises 20 percent of the meal, with 80 percent alkaline foods. Make your dough ahead of time and freeze it for the first-ever freezer pHizza dough!

Prep time: 10 minutes • **Cook time:** 12 minutes • **Yield:** 8 servings

Ingredients	Directions
Hold the Acids Pizza Dough (see recipe earlier in this section)	*1* Preheat oven to 425 degrees. Grease a 9-x-13 baking sheet with olive oil and top with pizza dough, spreading the dough gently to the edges by kneading it with your palms.
1 cup Pass the Pizza Sauce (see recipe earlier in this section)	
olive oil to grease baking sheet	*2* Bake the dough for 7 to 10 minutes. Remove it from the oven and let it rest for 1 minute.
½ cup sliced mushrooms	
½ eggplant, sliced thin	*3* Using a spatula, spread the pizza sauce evenly over the dough's surface, then layer the vegetables on top.
1 cup broccoli florets	
½ cup chopped red onion	*4* Sprinkle the mozzarella over the entire pizza and add the parmesan, if desired.
½ cup chopped zucchini	
1 tomato, seeded and diced	*5* Bake for 12 minutes, or until the cheese starts to brown at the edges and is completely melted.
1 cup fat-free mozzarella or soy cheese	
¼ cup grated parmesan (optional)	

Per serving: Calories 198 (From Fat 40); Fat 4g (Saturated 1g); Cholesterol 3mg; Sodium 754mg; Carbohydrate 35g; Dietary Fiber 9g; Protein 11g.

Padrón Pizza

Pepper lovers unite! If you've never had a Padrón pepper, boy, are you in for a treat. They look like baby bell peppers and are dark green. The majority of these Spanish gems have a mild, almost sweet flavor. However, about two out of ten pack quite a spicy punch (keeps life interesting). Serve this pizza with some chilled lemonade; the flavors pair nicely, and the citric acid can cool your burning taste buds.

You'll find Padrón peppers in the produce aisle of well-stocked grocery stores or at the local farmers' market when they're in season in your region. You can even order the seeds online and grow them yourself!

Prep time: 10 minutes • **Cook time:** 12 minutes • **Yield:** 8 servings

Ingredients	Directions
Hold the Acids Pizza Dough (see recipe earlier in this section)	**1** Preheat the oven to 425 degrees. Grease a 9-x-13 baking sheet with olive oil and spread the pizza dough on it.
2 teaspoons cold-pressed olive oil	**2** Pre-bake the dough for 7 to 10 minutes. Remove from the oven and set aside.
½ cup chopped red onion	
½ cup roasted garlic cloves	**3** Warm the olive oil in a large skillet over medium heat. Add the onion, garlic, and jalapeno, Padrón, and chili peppers. Sauté until the onions and peppers are tender — about 5 minutes. Remove from heat and set aside.
1 fresh jalapeno, sliced and seeded	
1 cup Padrón peppers, sliced	
2 red chili peppers, sliced	**4** Using a spatula, spread the pizza sauce evenly over the dough.
1 cup Pass the Pizza Sauce (see recipe earlier in this section)	**5** Layer the tomatoes on the pizza, followed by the onion-and-pepper mix. Sprinkle on the sea salt.
1 cup tomatoes, seeded and diced	
½ teaspoon sea salt	**6** Sprinkle the mozzarella and parmesan evenly over the pizza and bake for 12 minutes or until cheese is thoroughly melted and golden brown at the edges.
1 cup fat-free (skim) mozzarella or soy cheese	
¼ cup parmesan	

Per serving: Calories 201 (From Fat 49); Fat 5g (Saturated 1g); Cholesterol 3mg; Sodium 832mg; Carbohydrate 33g; Dietary Fiber 7g; Protein 10g.

Note: Turn on your stove's exhaust fan, and don't stand directly over the skillet while roasting the peppers. Oils are released into the steam, which can cause severe burning in your nose and eyes.

Capsaicinoids don't really hurt

Capsaicinoids are the natural chemical found in spicy plants that burn your mouth (or your eyes, if you rub them after chopping peppers). This chemical is an extremely alkaline oil, which latches onto your mucous membranes (lips, mouth, tongue, eyes) and stings like the devil. But it doesn't *really* hurt you — you are not actually burning off the first layer of your tongue, it just feels like it. These oily compounds bind with your pain receptors, making it feel as if the burning is a real tissue injury.

Ever see someone down a beer after a spicy burrito? Big mistake. The alcohol dilutes the alkaline oils and allows them to slip all over your mouth and down your esophagus, which equals even more burning pain everywhere. There's really only one thing you can do to alleviate the pepper pain; combat it with an acid. Next time you have a hot pepper eating contest, grab a couple lemon wedges first. The citric acid in the lemon will neutralize the alkaline oil in the pepper, and the fire in your tonsils will be quenched.

Savory Spinach Quichelets

If you enjoy lighter fare for dinner, this entrée is perfect. These egg-white tofu quichelets are a meal unto themselves, with a forkful of proteins and vegetables in each bite. This dish pairs nicely with grilled tomatoes, a spinach salad, or gazpacho. It's also delicious as pie filler, if you want to make your own crust using millet or spelt flour.

Prep time: 15 minutes • **Cook time:** 45 minutes • **Yield:** 12 muffins

Ingredients	Directions
3 tablespoons clarified butter, divided	*1* Preheat oven to 350 degrees. Grease a muffin tin with 1 tablespoon clarified butter or use paper liners.
1 10-ounce package frozen spinach, thawed and drained	*2* Place the remaining clarified butter, spinach, onion, scallions, mushrooms and garlic in a sauté pan. Cook over medium-low heat until the onions are translucent and the spinach is warmed.
1 yellow onion, diced	
¼ cup chopped scallions	
½ cup sliced mushrooms	
4 cloves garlic, pressed	*3* Place the egg whites and Tofutti Better Than Cream Cheese in a blender and mix on low speed until the mixture is creamy.
8 egg whites (or substitute)	
4 oz. Tofutti Better Than Cream Cheese	*4* In a large bowl (preferably one with a spout), mix all the ingredients thoroughly and add sea salt. Pour into muffin cups and bake for 25 minutes.
½ teaspoon sea salt	

Per serving: Calories 210 (From Fat 132); Fat 15g (Saturated 6g); Cholesterol 16mg; Sodium 588mg; Carbohydrate 10g; Dietary Fiber 3g; Protein 11g.

Lentil Pilaf

Besides the fact that it's oh so good for you, this dish will make you a rock star at the dinner table. Brace yourself for comments like, "When did you order takeout?" or "Did your mother make this?" You can use any kind of lentils in this dish, but I prefer the brown ones. They're easy to find, whereas red and green lentils are usually relegated to the health food stores.

Prep time: 15 minutes (plus 2 hours soaking time) • **Cook time:** 60 minutes • **Yield:** 4 to 6 servings

Ingredients	Directions
2 tablespoons cold-pressed olive oil	*1* Heat the olive oil in a small sauté pan over medium heat. Sauté the onion, garlic, and carrot for 5 minutes, or until the onion is translucent.
1 small yellow onion, diced	
1 small carrot, grated	
2 cloves garlic, chopped	*2* Add vegetable stock, sautéed vegetables, rice, lentils and remaining ingredients in a large pot, stir, and bring to a boil.
2 cups yeast-free vegetable stock	
1 cup wild rice	
½ cup brown lentils, rinsed	*3* Stir and reduce heat to a low simmer, cooking uncovered for 45 minutes. Remove and discard celery stalks.
1 teaspoon lemon juice	
1 celery stalk, halved lengthwise	*4* Salt and pepper to taste, stir, and add water as needed to keep pilaf moist.
1 tablespoon chopped parsley	
Sea salt and pepper to taste	

Per serving: Calories 326 (From Fat 73); Fat 8g (Saturated 1g); Cholesterol 0mg; Sodium 668mg; Carbohydrate 53g; Dietary Fiber 9g; Protein 14g.

Alkalinizing Poultry and Seafood

This is for the people struggling with their inner herbivore. If you're having difficulty dropping all the animal proteins as you transition to a plant-based diet, you can use these more carnivorous recipes.

Are you part mermaid? If so, you will be pleased to know that seafood packs a punch of healthy omega 3-fatty acids not found in other proteins. The good oily fishes (such as salmon) provide many healthy nutrients that can't be found in our two-legged food friends (such as chicken). Poultry and seafood are acidifying, but I show you how to combat that by making dishes loaded with vegetables and other alkalinizing ingredients.

Simply because you get to enjoy a little meat on the acid alkaline diet, don't go overboard. A serving of poultry or seafood is about the same size as the palm of your hand (thumb and fingers excluded). You don't want to consume more than that at a sitting.

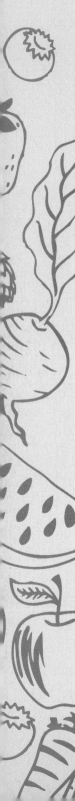

Chicken Hash

This farmer's dream is full of *umami,* that flavoring essence of meat that can't be captured using soy proteins. The chicken and potato leave an acidic ash during digestion; don't increase the amount of either if you adjust the recipe.

While you're at the grocery store, read the ground chicken labels. You want the real deal — not a ground-up mess including skin and fat. If you can't find anything suitable in the case, ask the butcher to grind up some pure chicken for you.

Prep time: 10 minutes • **Cook time:** 15 minutes • **Yield:** 4 servings

Ingredients	Directions
4 tablespoons cold-pressed olive oil, divided	*1* Grease a large nonstick skillet with 1 tablespoon of olive oil. Cook the chicken in the skillet over medium heat for 10 minutes, stirring frequently and breaking up any large clumps. Remove from heat and set aside.
12 ounces ground chicken	
½ cup diced yellow onion	
1 tablespoon grated carrot	*2* Grease skillet with 2 tablespoons of olive oil. Add the vegetables and cook them over low heat for 5 minutes, or until they're tender but not soggy.
½ cup shredded potato	
½ cup diced zucchini	
½ eggplant, peeled and chopped	*3* Stir the cooked chicken into the vegetable mixture in the skillet. Flatten with a nonstick spatula.
Sea salt and pepper to taste	
	4 Cook on medium for about 6 minutes. Resist the urge to stir.
	5 Drizzle the remaining olive oil on the top of the mixture and use a large, nonstick spatula to lift the hash and break it up into large chunks and flip them.
	6 Cook for another 6 minutes or until the desired crispiness is achieved.

Per serving: Calories 244 (From Fat 169); Fat 19g (Saturated 3g); Cholesterol 42mg; Sodium 185mg; Carbohydrate 9g; Dietary Fiber 2g; Protein 11g.

Salmon Fettuccini

Brace yourself for an eye-popping dose of garlic, butter, and omega 3-fatty acids all on one plate! Salmon is a cold-water fish, known for its beautiful pink coloring and very non-fishy taste. Get choosy about your salmon selection, picking only fish labeled "wild caught" or better yet, "wild Alaskan," which are not farmed and have no ingredients other than what is natural. I'm not a big fan of the "organic" kind, as the term is used pretty loosely when it comes to fish (varying degrees of regulation depending on your location).

Prep time: 15 minutes • **Cook time:** 15 minutes • **Yield:** 4 to 6 servings

Ingredients	*Directions*
12 ounces fresh salmon, cut into filets	*1* Wash salmon and keep the skin intact. Pre heat oiled grill to medium.
Sea salt and pepper to taste	
1 tablespoon clarified butter	*2* Salt and pepper salmon filet to taste, grill for 6 minutes, skin side down, and flip. Grill for another 6 minutes, or until the meat flakes off easily with a fork.
Juice of one lemon, about 3 tablespoons	
2 cloves garlic, minced	*3* In a small pan, heat butter, lemon juice, and garlic over medium heat. Stir and cook for 3 minutes.
12 ounces spelt fettuccini, cooked	
20 spinach leaves	*4* Remove skin from salmon and divide into large flakes, or chunks of meat. Toss with warm pasta, garlic-butter sauce, spinach, and fresh basil.
2 tablespoons finely chopped fresh basil, or 1 tablespoon dried	

Per serving: Calories 524 (From Fat 108); Fat 12g (Saturated 3g); Cholesterol 62mg; Sodium 233mg; Carbohydrate 76g; Dietary Fiber 10g; Protein 35g.

Tip: Don't discard the lemon after juicing it. Slice the rind into wedges and place them in a small bowl on the counter. The odor helps combat any fishy smell the salmon leaves in your kitchen.

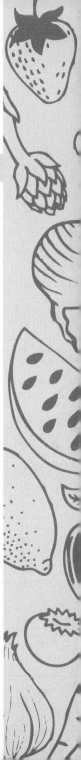

Seafood Combo

Shrimp and scallops make up this herbed seafood dish. You can buy shrimp and scallops frozen or fresh — it depends on how close you live to the water (and if you'd want to eat seafood out of your local waterways). The smaller the scallop, the more tender it is. Conversely, I have found smaller shrimps, although tender, tend to taste like brine and fish. So, go for the jumbos when it comes to shrimp — and enjoy the jumbo shrimp oxymoron.

Prep time: 25 minutes • **Cook time**: 20 minutes • **Yield:** 4 to 6 servings

Ingredients	Directions
4 tablespoons clarified butter, divided	**1** In a small saucepan, heat 2 tablespoons of the clarified butter and sauté the garlic, scallions, and green bell peppers over medium heat. Cook for 5 minutes, or until green peppers are tender but still crunchy. Pour in the vegetable broth and reduce heat to low. Cook until the broth evaporates and set aside.
1 clove garlic, minced or pressed	
½ cup chopped scallions	
½ cup green bell peppers, seeded and diced	**2** Cook pasta according to package directions and set aside.
½ cup vegetable broth	
1 pound jumbo raw shrimp, peeled and de-veined	**3** Steam broccoli in the microwave by adding ¼ cup water to a microwave-safe bowl and cooking on high for 1 minute. Drain any remaining water and set aside.
¾ pound small bay scallops	
3 tablespoons chopped basil	**4** In a small pot, bring soy milk to a low boil. Slowly stir in spelt flour, stirring often until thickened. Add diced tomatoes and reduce heat to a simmer for 5 minutes. Stir and remove from heat.
2 tablespoons chopped parsley	
1 teaspoon marjoram	
1 cup broccoli florets	**5** In a skillet, heat the remaining 2 tablespoons of clarified butter over medium heat. Add shrimp, scallops, basil, parsley, and marjoram. Gently stir and cook, uncovered, for about 3 minutes, or until the seafood is cooked (longer if the shrimp and scallops are frozen).
½ cup soy milk	
2 tablespoons spelt flour	
2 cups diced tomatoes	
12 ounces cooked spelt or vegetable pasta	**6** Toss all ingredients together with cooked pasta and serve warm. Garnish with fresh cracked black pepper if desired.

Per serving: Calories 668 (From Fat 164); Fat 18g (Saturated 8g); Cholesterol 257mg; Sodium 602mg; Carbohydrate 75g; Dietary Fiber 11g; Protein 56g.

Chapter 16

Snacks: Keeping the Belly Happy

In This Chapter

▶ Stop starving yourself

▶ Blending up goodness

▶ Satiating and slimming snacks

▶ Snacking on pH-friendly treats

1 once embarked on a trendy fad diet (don't ask, I won't tell). I read the books, gathered the cooking supplies, and felt ready to start. Exactly one night into the diet after a scant meal that didn't fulfill either of us, my husband asked, "So, what can we snack on?" If you're like me and enjoy grazing throughout the day, this chapter is the one for you.

It's important that you stay *satiated* — full, satisfied, and happy — otherwise, it's too easy to grab a crunchy vending machine snack or buy those candy bars from your coworker. It's your lucky day — in this chapter, I tell you exactly why you should snack — and snack a lot.

Stop Starving Yourself

Anyone on a diet that severely restricts calories will turn purple at this news: Your metabolism slows down, and you may become more irritable when you starve yourself. We all have an inner caveman who likes to speak up when he thinks he's being starved. Your body slows down all processes and goes into what is known as *starvation mode* in which it hoards all calories and fat for what it thinks is a long stretch of no food.

Your inner caveman may awaken and start hoarding after as little as six food-less hours, or as long as one day; the rate your body hoards fats and calories is different for everyone. It's dependent on how fast — or slow — your metabolism functions.

Aim to eat five to six small meals daily to keep your metabolism at peak performance. A meal doesn't have to mean a four-course entrée — a satisfying snack can fill the requirement.

Eating healthy snacks every few hours keeps your metabolism running at peak performance and stops the bingeing sessions later in the day. It also stops your body from producing excess acids while trying to support your brain with the energy it needs to function. So I say again, "Snack away!"

Grass is good

There's a reason those farm animals look so healthy and happy (besides the fact that they don't have bosses, mortgages — or thumbs, for that matter): grass is good. But you need to choose the right grass — don't go munching on your Bermuda out back or your neighbors will think you've lost your mind. If you want to experiment with your own Power Greens recipe, consider adding these consumable grasses:

- Barley grass
- Oat grass
- Wheat grass
- Kelp (sea grass)

Soy Surprise

A word on blenders — you get what you pay for. My first blender, a wedding present, leaked all over my counter the first time I tried to pulse ice. If you don't already have one, consider buying a blender with the attachment you can use as a drinking cup after blending your smoothie (how convenient is that).

Prep time: 5 minutes • **Yield**: 3 servings

Ingredients	Directions
1 cup vanilla soy yogurt **2 tablespoons soy powder**	**1** Put the yogurt, soy powder, milk, and barley powder into the blender and mix well for about 1 minute.
½ cup almond milk **1 tablespoon barley grass powder**	**2** Slowly add the ice and pulse on High to mix.
1 cup crushed ice, or 6 cubes **½ banana**	**3** Add the remaining ingredients and mix until everything is blended. Add water, one tablespoon at a time, as needed if the mixture is too thick.
1-gram packet Stevia, or ¼ teaspoon powder, or 6 drops liquid, or ½ teaspoon minced fresh leaves	
4 ounces silken tofu	
Dash vanilla extract	

Per serving: Calories 121 (From Fat 23); Fat 3g (Saturated 0g); Cholesterol 0mg; Sodium 100mg; Carbohydrate 16g; Dietary Fiber 2g; Protein 10g.

Power Greens

Don't let the color put you off — just imagine you're drinking your salad and meeting your five-a-day veggie needs in one delicious concoction. This smoothie is exploding with antioxidants, vitamins, and minerals — not to mention taste. For the newbie smoothie consumer, you can start with the basic blend of tofu and apples, adding one type of green at a time.

Prep time: 5 minutes • **Yield**: 3 servings

Ingredients	*Directions*
½ **cup raw spinach leaves, stems trimmed off**	*1* In a blender, mix the spinach, broccoli, ice cubes, and aloe vera juice thoroughly.
¼ **cup broccoli florets**	
4 ice cubes	*2* Add the tofu, carrot juice, barley grass powder, and garlic.
¼ **cup aloe vera juice**	
4 ounces silken tofu	*3* Add apple juice, one tablespoon at a time, if the mixture is too thick to drink.
½ **cup carrot juice, natural and unsweetened**	
1 tablespoon barley grass powder	
1 tablespoon garlic powder	
¼ **cup apple juice, unsweetened organic**	

Per serving: Calories 91 (From Fat 13); Fat 1g (Saturated 0g); Cholesterol 0mg; Sodium 35mg; Carbohydrate 17g; Dietary Fiber 3g; Protein 4g.

Rooty Tooty Smoothie

The Rooty Tooty rounds out my smoothie recipe collection with a beta carotene, vitamin C, and potassium punch. This smoothie tastes best on crisp autumn mornings — but you can enjoy it anytime of the year by stocking up on pie pumpkins when they're in season, then cooking and freezing them. (See the nearby "Cooking your own pumpkin" sidebar for tips.)

Of course, you have year-round access to canned pumpkin as well, but I prefer to use the real thing in this recipe. If you use the canned stuff, just be sure it's unsweetened.

Prep time: 5 minutes • **Yield**: 3 servings

Ingredients	Directions
½ **cup cooked sweet potatoes, in small chunks**	*1* In a blender, mix the sweet potatoes and almond milk thoroughly.
½ **cup unsweetened almond milk**	
½ **cup carrot juice, unsweetened**	*2* Add the carrot juice, pumpkin, stevia, cinnamon, and allspice, and mix thoroughly.
½ **cup cooked pumpkin**	
1 1-gram packet stevia, or ¼ **teaspoon powder, or 6 drops liquid, or** ½ **teaspoon fresh, minced leaves**	*3* Add more water, one tablespoon at a time, if mixture is too thick to drink.
1 teaspoon cinnamon	
½ **teaspoon allspice**	

Per serving: Calories 53 (From Fat 6); Fat 1g (Saturated 0g); Cholesterol 0mg; Sodium 49mg, Carbohydrate 12g; Dietary Fiber 2g; Protein 1g.

Kale Chips

Everyone needs a good, crunchy snack to pair with the dips in this chapter. These chips provide your answer to a guilt-free, alkalinizing snack. Bitter when raw, kale leaves can be dehydrated or baked to make crispy snacks. Store them in little plastic baggies for easy access.

Prep time: 5 minutes • **Cook time:** 15 minutes • **Yield:** 3 servings

Ingredients	Directions
5 fresh kale leaves **2 tablespoons cold-pressed olive oil** **1 teaspoon sea salt**	**1** Preheat the oven to 325 degrees. If the kale leaves are still attached to the tough stems, cut the leaves off and discard the stems. Wash and dry the leaves.
	2 Using kitchen scissors, cut the kale leaves into bite-sized pieces. Place in a large, resealable plastic baggie.
	3 Add the olive oil and salt; shake the bag until the kale is thoroughly coated. You may need to add a little more olive oil, one tablespoon at a time, if your leaves are huge.
	4 Line a baking sheet with parchment paper and spread the kale leaves in a single layer. Bake for 15 minutes or until the edges of each "chip" start to brown.

Per serving: Calories 136 (From Fat 88); Fat 10g (Saturated 1g); Cholesterol 0mg; Sodium 816mg; Carbohydrate 11g; Dietary Fiber 2g; Protein 4g.

Note: Add one teaspoon of garlic powder for a tangier chip.

Dipping Makes It Fun

I have two small children who actually eat their fruits and vegetables . . . un-coerced! How do I work such magic, you might ask? I keep their fruit and vegetable platters fun by adding different dips and constantly experimenting. Dips make otherwise boring raw produce acceptable as an appetizer or even a dish to share at your next block party.

Store-bought dips just won't do when you're balancing your pH. My recipes exchange the acidifying sour creams and cheeses for things like mashed veggies or soy yogurt. Only the acids are left out, not the taste.

I include *Tofutti's Better Than Cream Cheese* in many recipes, but don't read it as an endorsement or a sales pitch — it's just what I use. Feel free to exchange it for another cream cheese replacement product if you wish; there are a few different types on the market.

Blenderizing up a storm

Honestly, what *can't* you put in the blender? I once ground up steak for a patient who had difficulty swallowing and made him a steak-shake (I don't encourage it). If your blender is hiding in the kitchen cabinet, it's time to dust that puppy off and give it a spot of honor on the counter.

Smoothies have regained popularity as both a health food and an easy meal. Pick a little protein, add a couple fruits or veggies, and you have a delicious, drinkable meal. Some smoothie tips to consider:

✔ Soy powder, silken tofu, or whey powder provide protein

✔ Ice, water, moist fruits and veggies (cucumber, pumpkin, watermelon), and non-sweetened fruit juices thin the smoothie

✔ Add spices — garlic for greens, cinnamon for fruits — to keep it interesting

✔ If the spinach leaves are just spinning in the blender, try bunching up a few into a small ball and adding them with a harder vegetable, like carrots

✔ Make your own spicy tomato-based drink with tomatoes, carrots, bell peppers, and cayenne pepper

---

Dad's Dilly Dip

Fast, easy, and it pairs with everything — I'll bet Dilly Dip becomes a standard item in your fridge. Use fresh-squeezed lemon juice for the best flavor, and consider adding some lemon zest if you want even more alkalines.

Prep time: 5 minutes • **Yield**: 4 to 6 servings

Ingredients	Directions
1 cup plain soy yogurt **4 ounces Tofutti Better Than Cream Cheese** **1 tablespoon lemon juice** **2 tablespoons dried chives** **2 tablespoons dried dill weed** **½ teaspoon sea salt** **Dash pepper**	*1* In a blender or food processor mix the yogurt, cream cheese, and lemon juice until smooth. *2* Stir in the chives, dill, salt, and pepper. Refrigerate overnight for the best flavor, or chill for one hour before serving.

Per serving: Calories 120 (From Fat 79); Fat 9g (Saturated 2g); Cholesterol 0mg; Sodium 435mg; Carbohydrate 9g; Dietary Fiber 1g; Protein 3g.

Don't dis dill, dry it!

Dill, also called dill weed, is an amazingly versatile herb. It has a flavor unlike anything else, and is tasty in soups, salads, breads, dips, seafood dishes, and — of course — pickles. This weed-like (hence the loving name dill *weed*) herb grows out of control — regardless if your thumb is green or not. It's pretty hard to kill dill, which makes this herb a great starter plant for the would-be gardener (just don't try to transplant it, *that* never ends well).

You can use either the seeds or the dill leaves in cooking. Fresh dill imparts a much stronger taste to the dish, which is why I personally use dried dill. I find the fresh kind just a teensy bit overpowering. Drying dill only takes a few days:

1. Cut off portions of the plant to dry (or take it all if your first frost is near).

2. Loop twine or a rubber band around the bottom of the stalk (or stalks, if drying more than one).

3. Hang them upside down for five to seven days in a warm, dry area out of direct sunlight.

4 Break off the leaves or crumble the flowers for later use. Store in an airtight container.

Chili Dip

Sssh — don't tell anyone that sometimes I make a meal out of this delicious dip. The lentils and rice stick to your ribs and will satisfy even the heartiest snackers. I eat this dip during my "it's midnight and I'm craving cold pizza" moments as a healthier substitute.

Prep time: 5 minutes • **Yield**: 4 to 6 servings

Ingredients	Directions
12 ounces cooked lentils	**1** Warm the lentils and vegetable broth in a small sauce-pan. Add the onions, bell pepper, garlic, and tomatoes. Cook over medium heat for 8 minutes or until the onions are tender.
¼ cup yeast-free vegetable broth	
¼ cup chopped onion	
¼ cup chopped green bell pepper	**2** Blend the Tofutti Better Than Cream Cheese, chili powder, cumin, and sea salt in a blender or food processor until smooth.
½ clove garlic, pressed	
1 cup diced tomatoes	
2 ounces Tofutti Better Than Cream Cheese	**3** In a large bowl, mix the rice with the cream cheese blend and lentil vegetable mix, and stir thoroughly. Serve warm.
½ tablespoon chili powder	
½ teaspoon cumin	
¼ teaspoon sea salt	
Dash paprika	
½ cup cooked wild rice	

Per serving: Calories 181 (From Fat 44); Fat 5g (Saturated 1g); Cholesterol 0mg; Sodium 435mg; Carbohydrate 27g; Dietary Fiber 8g; Protein 10g.

Note: Scoop up mouthfuls with some fresh kale chips, focaccia, or a spoon (I won't tell). A focaccia recipe is disguised as pizza dough in Chapter 15.

Pumpkin Pie Dip

In my household, pumpkin pie is not relegated to holidays or fall festivals. Keep a couple cans of pumpkin (hold the syrup, please, just get plain pumpkin) on hand so you can make this dip or the Rooty Tooty smoothie whenever the mood strikes you.

Prep time: 5 minutes • **Yield**: 4 to 6 servings

Ingredients	Directions
8 ounces Tofutti Better Than Cream Cheese	**1** Using a mixer, whip the Tofutti Better Than Cream Cheese and canned pumpkin until smooth.
15 ounces unsweetened canned pumpkin	
1 teaspoon cinnamon	**2** Add the cinnamon, allspice, nutmeg, and pecans, and stir until mixed. Chill in the refrigerator for one hour before serving.
¼ teaspoon allspice	
¼ teaspoon nutmeg	
10 pecans, smashed	

Per serving: Calories 227 (From Fat 172); Fat 19g (Saturated 4g); Cholesterol 0mg; Sodium 275mg; Carbohydrate 12g; Dietary Fiber 6g; Protein 4g.

Note: Cut a cooked sweet potato in half lengthwise and top with this dip for a hearty alkalinizing snack.

Cooking your own pumpkin

Pumpkins are a seasonal vegetable, usually harvested before the first frost. Most of the time, if you want pumpkin, you use canned pumpkin, because these squashes have a very narrow harvesting window. However, when those glorious orange globes make their appearance in the grocery store, you can be ready to make (and freeze for later) your own cooked pumpkin:

1. Use a sharp knife to cut the top off of the pumpkin.

2. Use a sturdy spoon (or your hands) to scoop out the seeds and stringy pumpkin guts. Set aside.

3. Chop remaining pumpkin into quarters, peel, and then cut into two-inch cubes.

4. Fill a large pot with water, add the pumpkin cubes and a pinch of sea salt.

5. Boil the pumpkin for 35 minutes or until a fork easily mashes a piece of pumpkin.

6. Drain and mash by hand or in a blender. Store in the freezer in an airtight container.

Don't toss those seeds! Separate them from the gooey pumpkin innards by washing in a colander. Toss them with some cold-pressed olive oil, spread them on a baking sheet, salt them, and roast them at 275 degrees for two hours or until they're crunchy. Yum!

Fruity Dip

Instead of drowning those healthy fruit slices in sugar or syrup, consider using this delicious low-cal dip. You can toss this dip with a bowl of chopped fruit for a homemade fruit salad — you'll love this refreshingly cool and sweet snack when that summer heat kicks in.

Prep time: 5 minutes • **Yield**: 2 servings

Ingredients	Directions
2 ounces Tofutti Better Than Cream Cheese 2 tablespoons honey ¼ cup squeezed orange juice ½ teaspoon ground cinnamon	**1** In a blender or food processor mix all the ingredients until they're smooth and creamy. Chill for one hour before use.

Per serving: Calories 160 (From Fat 74); Fat 8g (Saturated 2g); Cholesterol 0mg; Sodium 136mg; Carbohydrate 22g; Dietary Fiber 0g; Protein 1g.

Tip: Add soy or almond milk, one tablespoon at a time, for a thinner dip. This thinned dip works great as a dressing for a fruit salad.

Satiating Simple Snacks

If it's weight control you're seeking, these satiating simples will fill up your belly without stretching your waistline. I'll give you some unsolicited calorie-control advice: If your stomach feels full, you won't be tempted to eat high-calorie foods.

I've tried some pretty wild diets in my day, but none of them whittled my waistline like this simple tip: I zap a mug of vegetable broth in the microwave and drink it whenever I feel like snacking. The warm broth tricks my stomach into thinking it's full, and my brain stops sending the "feed me" signals — you know, the ones that make your stomach groan and make disgusting noises at mealtime.

Making banana "ice"

This trick is so simple and so delicious that I should copyright it (oops, guess I just did). I like to add banana ice to fresh juices, smoothies, or stir it up with soy yogurt for some added natural sweetness. All you need is an ice cube tray and some fresh bananas (I don't like brown spots on my "ice"). Slice up the bananas into half-inch chunks and place one piece in each ice cube slot. Freeze and use like ice.

Mashed "Taters"

Mashed cauliflower is so filling, so delicious, and so not my original idea. I'm not sure what culinary genius coined this one, but over the years I've made it my own and tricked many a dinner guest with its deliciousness (they thought they were getting potatoes).

Prep time: 10 minutes • **Cook time:** 30 minutes • **Yield:** 4 servings

Ingredients	Directions
1 head cauliflower 8 cups water ¼ cup almond milk ¼ cup clarified butter, warmed ½ teaspoon sea salt ¼ teaspoon paprika Dash pepper Fresh chopped parsley sprigs (optional)	*1* Preheat the oven to 325 degrees. Wash and dry the cauliflower, then chop it into pieces, discarding the core and tough stems. *2* Boil the cauliflower in water for 20 to 25 minutes, or until you can easily mash a floret with a fork. Drain the water. *3* Put the cauliflower and almond milk in a mixing bowl and beat on low. *4* Slowly pour in the clarified butter, then add the salt, paprika, and pepper, and continue mixing until all the ingredients are blended. Scoop into an oven-safe baking dish. *5* Bake for 10 minutes and serve hot. Garnish with fresh parsley, if desired.

Per serving: Calories 152 (From Fat 119); Fat 13g (Saturated 8g); Cholesterol 033mg; Sodium 341mg; Carbohydrate 8g; Dietary Fiber 4g; Protein 3g.

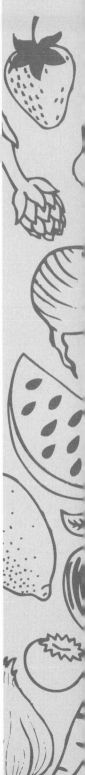

Holy Guacamole

It's a dip, it's a spread, no — it's Holy Guacamole! Why is it holy, you ask? Because the taste is divine, and the avocado and lemon are two of the most alkalinizing fruits out there. Not to mention — what *can't* you spread guacamole on?

Prep time: 10 minutes • **Yield**: 6 servings

Ingredients	Directions
2 ripe avocados, pitted	**1** In a small bowl, mash the avocadoes with a potato masher.
1 small tomato, seeded and finely chopped	
½ tablespoon fresh lime juice	**2** Stir the remaining ingredients into the mashed avocados and serve immediately.
½ small yellow onion, finely chopped	
2 garlic cloves, pressed	
¼ teaspoon sea salt	
Dash of pepper	
Minced fresh cilantro leaf	

Per serving: Calories 97 (From Fat 76); Fat 8g (Saturated 2g); Cholesterol 0mg; Sodium 97mg; Carbohydrate 6g; Dietary Fiber 5g; Protein 1g.

Tip: Use Holy Guacamole as a topping in place of recipes that call for cheese, butter, or mayonnaise spreads. It pairs wonderfully with the Zucchini Quesadillas (recipe in Chapter 15), works well on a sandwich, or as a standalone snack served with kale chips (see the recipe earlier in this chapter).

Tackling the avocado

The amazing avocado — the only fruit full of omega 3-fatty acids. It's believed that omega 3-fatty acids can help protect you from cardiovascular disease. These fatty acids are *essential nutrients*, which means that you must eat them, your body cannot make them. The one caveat is that avocados are ripe with calories, and even though they're good calories, they're still calories.

Avocadoes are covered with a thick black or green skin, which protects the soft, creamy fruit inside. Gently squeeze the avocado to check for ripeness. You should be able to indent the fruit if it is ripe (if you crush it with a gentle squeeze it is probably over-ripe).

The first time I peeled an avocado was the last time I ate one for years. Worse than a kiwi, peeling an avocado is a messy process that ends up making you toss half the fruit with the peel. I have a better way:

1. Thoroughly wash and dry the avocado.

2. Using a sharp kitchen knife, slice the fruit length-wise, pushing the knife all the way to the large seed in the center.

3. Grab both halves of the avocado and gently twist them apart. Set aside the seedless half.

4. Put the half with the remaining seed on a cutting board. With a chopping motion, embed the blade of a very sharp knife horizontally in the hard seed. Give a twist and the seed pops out on the knife!

5. Use a large spoon to gently scoop the fruit out of its shell halves.

Avocadoes ripen quickly without their protective shell, so use it soon or refrigerate it.

After-School or In-Office Treats

Although chopped fruits and vegetables satisfy your hunger *and* keep your pH on the alkaline side of the scale, telling you to eat them would make for a pretty *boring* chapter on snacks. These recipes work as a great after-school snack to enjoy with the kids or pack nicely for the office.

Beggars Popcorn

Although as a vegetable corn forms an acidic ash in your digestive tract, popcorn is a fairly neutral food — so I paired it with some alkalizing spices to keep your pH on track. I'm not a physicist, so you'll have to experiment with your microwave cooking time and power level. (I have a button that says "popcorn" — love it!)

Prep time: 5 minutes • **Cook time:** 2 - 5 minutes • **Yield:** About 4 cups popped

Ingredients	Directions
2 tablespoons popcorn kernels **2 bursts nonstick cooking spray** **Cinnamon to taste** **Chili powder to taste** **Cayenne pepper to taste** **Garlic powder to taste** **1 teaspoon sea salt**	*1* Place the uncooked popcorn in a brown paper bag. Spray the inside of the bag and kernels with nonstick cooking spray and fold the top of the bag down about five times tightly, leaving plenty of room for popped corn. *2* Microwave on medium-high for about 2 minutes (or until popping slows down to 3 seconds between pops). *3* Sprinkle with the cinnamon, chili powder, cayenne, garlic, and sea salt. Re-close the bag and give it a good shake.

Per 1 cup serving: Calories 32 (From Fat 4); Fat 0g (Saturated 0g); Cholesterol 0mg; Sodium 576mg; Carbohydrate 7g; Dietary Fiber 1g; Protein 1g.

Lemonade by the glass

I talk about the power of hydration in Chapter 6 and the beauty of lemons in Chapter 2; so how can you best use this information? By drinking lemonade by the glass, of course. The water carries that lemon juice (and pulp) down your digestive tract, where it forms an alkalizing ash just waiting to combat any acids you've eaten today.

I'm far too lazy to sit and cut 20 lemons (or open 20 packets of Stevia) at once, but when the craving calls, I like to have a nice, chilled glass of lemonade. Here's how to make just one glass:

1. Wash a lemon and cut half of it into wedges, get rid of the seeds.

2. Fill an eight-ounce glass half-full with water.

3. Squeeze the lemon (hard, get some of that pulp in there, too) into the water.

4. Add one packet of Stevia and stir.

5. Pour the lemonade over ice and enjoy! If you're the fancy type, stick a sprig of fresh mint on the rim of a chilled glass.

Scrumptious Salsa

Salsa on focaccia, salsa on Stuffed Green Peppers, salsa on Spinach Quiche . . . do I need to go on? I'd put salsa on my salsa, if that wasn't such a cliché. It gets watery after sitting in the fridge for a few days, so I like to make it and eat it right away. (I don't usually see any Scrumptious Salsa leftovers anyway — it's too good!)

Prep time: 10 minutes • **Yield**: 4 servings

Ingredients	Directions
4 medium tomatoes, peeled and diced	1 Mix all the ingredients together either using a food processor (for a creamier texture) or by hand (for a rougher, crunchier salsa).
¼ cup chopped red onion	
Jalapeno pepper, seeded and finely chopped	2 Garnish with fresh parsley and serve chilled with Kale Chips. (See recipe earlier in this chapter — make them bigger than what's called for if you want to scoop up the salsa.)
1 tablespoon cold-pressed olive oil	
1 teaspoon sea salt	
1 teaspoon cumin	
1 teaspoon minced garlic	
Fresh parsley (optional)	

Per serving: Calories 73 (From Fat 36); Fat 4g (Saturated 1g); Cholesterol 0mg; Sodium 582mg; Carbohydrate 9g; Dietary Fiber 1g; Protein 1g.

Almond Roast

You'll be stashing these suckers away like a squirrel in late October. Not only are they natural sources of calcium, almonds are one of the few nuts that are very alkalinizing. Next time you're headed to the movies or a ball game, consider bringing a big bag of these roasted goodies.

Prep time: 5 minutes • **Cook time**: 30 minutes • **Yield**: 4 to 6 servings

Ingredients	Directions
2 cups raw almonds	*1* Preheat the oven to 275 degrees. Place the almonds in a large, resealable plastic bag. Pour olive oil into the bag and shake it well.
¼ cup cold-pressed olive oil	
1 teaspoon sea salt	
2 1-gram packets of Stevia, or ½ teaspoon powdered, or 12 drops of liquid, or 1 teaspoon fresh, minced leaves	*2* Spread the almonds onto an ungreased baking sheet.
	3 Mix stevia and salt in a small bowl. Sprinkle it over the almonds and bake them for 30 minutes, stirring once during baking.

Per serving: Calories 545 (From Fat 444); Fat 49g (Saturated 4g); Cholesterol 0mg; Sodium 575mg; Carbohydrate 14g; Dietary Fiber 9g; Protein 15g.

Filling up on fiber

Most people need between 25 and 35 grams of fiber each day. Makes you think twice about getting excited when that ad quotes, "two *whole* grams of fiber in each serving," because you're going to have to eat about 12 servings to meet the minimum RDA (recommended daily allowance) of fiber.

This nutrient is like the sponge to your colon — it sweeps it out and keeps it clean. A high-fiber diet is linked to decreased bad cholesterol levels, less heart disease, and it may even lower your risk for several cancers, such as colon cancer. It also helps with weight management — fiber fills the belly.

Fact is, you'll probably have very little problem meeting your daily fiber requirements on the acid alkaline diet. The best natural source of fiber is found in fruits and vegetables — they are a complete source of both *soluble* (dissolves in water, slightly digestible) and *insoluble* (absolutely not digestible — think corn) fiber.

If you're still wanting more of this nutrient, try keeping the peels on your fruits and veggies. Obviously I'm not talking about inedible peels like a banana, but the fruits and vegetables that have edible peels, such as sweet potatoes.

Terrific Tomatoes

Bookmark this page if you are frequently invited to events that require a dish from home — you can thank me later. Quinoa is a very versatile grain, which can be enjoyed hot or cold and does not acidify your pH. In this dish, it takes on a salad-like quality and cuts down the acidity (pH-wise, pre-digestion) of the tomatoes.

Prep time: 10 minutes • **Cook time:** 15 minutes • **Yield:** 10 to 12 servings

Ingredients	Directions
36 cherry tomatoes	*1* Wash and dry the cherry tomatoes. Cut ¼ inch off the stem side and discard; cut ⅛ inch off the bottoms and line them up on a baking tray. Use a small spoon to remove the seeds and pulp, which you discard.
1 cup quinoa	
1 and ½ cups water	
½ cup finely chopped snow peas	*2* Rinse the quinoa using a fine colander or wire mesh strainer. Place the grain in a medium saucepan, cover it with water, and bring to a boil.
2 tablespoons cold-pressed olive oil	
1 teaspoon cilantro	*3* Reduce the heat to a low simmer and cover the pot tightly. Cook for 15 minutes, then set the pot aside and let the quinoa cool.
2 tablespoons lemon juice	
4 scallions, chopped	
	4 Steam the snow peas in a microwave-safe bowl with a dash of water for about 1 minute, or until crisp-tender. Set aside.
	5 Mix the olive oil, cilantro, and lemon juice in a small bowl, set aside.
	6 Mix the cooked quinoa, snow peas, and olive oil mix thoroughly. Spoon mixture into tomatoes, overflowing a little at the top. Garnish with the chopped scallions.

Per serving: Calories 102 (From Fat 48); Fat 5g (Saturated 1g); Cholesterol 0mg; Sodium 13mg; Carbohydrate 13g; Dietary Fiber 2g; Protein 2g.

Pizza Cups

All you have to do is say the word "pizza" and I start salivating. Make the dough ahead of time and these will cook in a jiffy. (Find the recipe for Hold the Acids Pizza Dough in Chapter 15.) I don't want to sauté sauce all day for a simple snack, so I use a commercial sugar-free, gluten-free brand of spaghetti sauce called Bove's. (You can find it in most well-stocked grocery stores or online at http://boves.com.)

Prep time: 15 minutes • **Cook time**: 15 minutes • **Yield**: 6 to 8 servings

Ingredients	Directions
2 tablespoons cold-pressed olive oil	**1** Preheat the oven to 375 degrees. Grease two muffin pans with olive oil.
Home-made pizza dough, divided (see Chapter 13 for the recipe)	**2** Roll dough on a floured surface to about ½ inch uniform thickness.
1 tablespoon spelt or millet flour	**3** Use a small glass, such as a juice glass, to cut out two-inch circles (or thereabouts) from dough. Place each cut-out piece of dough in a greased muffin tin.
1 cup sugar-free, gluten-free spaghetti or pizza sauce	
½ cup minced onion	
1 tablespoon oregano	**4** Place one spoonful of sauce on top of each piece of dough. Sprinkle with onion, oregano, basil and mozzarella or soy cheese.
1 tablespoon basil	
1 cup no-fat mozzarella or soy cheese	**5** Bake for 10 to 15 minutes, or until crusts are golden.

Per serving: Calories 288 (From Fat 111); Fat 12g (Saturated 2g); Cholesterol 4mg; Sodium 910mg; Carbohydrate 38g; Dietary Fiber 9g; Protein 13g.

Chapter 17

Delicious Desserts

*E*ating dessert is where following an acid alkaline diet gets tricky. Almost anything you purchase in the bakery is a pH no-no. Refined flour, whole eggs, cream, and sugar all acidify your pH. So what *can* you eat for dessert? Have no fear, your dessert queen is here. You can still eat the occasional yummy treats you enjoy by keeping the proper pH exchanges in mind. I show you how in this chapter.

Foods to Run Away From

Get your sneakers laced up, it's time to run away from any dessert containing:

✔ Dairy

✔ Refined flour

✔ Sugar

✔ Whole eggs

This list probably encapsulates all those bakery pastries (especially the ones with the cream filling). I'm not saying you have to skip eating your brother's wedding cake or bake your son a spinach quiche for his birthday, but on a daily basis, it's better to avoid these common baking and dessert ingredients. As a whole, they are very acidifying and will wreck your pH-balancing efforts.

You can continue to enjoy dessert occasionally on a pH balanced diet, but it requires some exchanges and knowledge of what baking ingredients impact your pH.

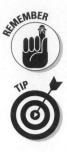

Dessert should be an occasional treat. Eating dessert every single day and maintaining a healthy, alkaline lifestyle are as comparable as sitting on the couch and growing a six-pack of abdominal muscles — they just don't go together. I suffer a sweet tooth, and I know firsthand how those little bite-sized candies add up throughout the day (as do the mini donut holes from the office kitchen).

Consider these ways to stop over-indulging in desserts:

- ✔ Write down every sweet you put in your mouth in one day, including sodas, shakes, and other drinkable desserts.

- ✔ Consider why you need the sweets — are you hungry? Tired? Want the sugar pick-me-up?

- ✔ Eat a piece of fruit, drink a glass of lemon water, or pop a piece of sugar-free gum in your mouth to satisfy your craving for something sweet.

- ✔ Get busy doing something else. Take a walk, finish a project — many times, snacking on sweets provides a false psychological comfort when what you're really doing it avoiding an unpleasant task.

Embracing Baked Goods

It's not as terrible as it sounds — an exchange here, a swap there, and before you know it, you're back to enjoying tasty desserts that won't impact your pH.

I've been saving up this news until right now: If you want a *bite* of an acidifying dessert — go ahead. As long as it's not daily, just a bite of a scrumptious chocolate bakery concoction may be enough to satisfy your sweet tooth, helping you avoid the overindulgences that accompany self-deprivation. (But I still think you should avoid those yellow cream-filled thingies — no one really knows what they're made of anyway.)

Refined flours

You have options when it comes to dessert recipes containing flour. By discovering how to make delicious desserts without all the acidifying ingredients, you remain in control of your pH without suffering a life of no treats. Instead of wheat or white refined flour, try baking with:

- ✔ Almond flour (also known as almond meal)
- ✔ Millet flour
- ✔ Spelt flour

What the heck is stevia?

First and foremost, stevia is an herb. Also known as *sweet leaf,* stevia is a natural sugar alternative, not a manufactured chemical molecule like the artificial sweeteners. Before discovering stevia, I downed those artificial sweeteners like a mouse in the laboratory — but not anymore. Stevia leaves are hundreds of times sweeter than sugar, but virtually calorie free! Many of my recipes call for stevia — from smoothies to dips — because it has a negligible impact on your pH and blood sugar levels, unlike its cousin sugar cane.

Stevia comes in single-use packets, a powder, and liquid concentrates. Avoid the crystallized stevias, which are usually a combination of sucralose (which acidifies) and stevia. Reach for the powdered, liquid, or natural version. You can grow stevia and use the raw leaves (dried or fresh) in any of the recipes calling for stevia.

Wait, there's even more choices to make . . . some brands of the liquid concentrate come in flavors that include apricot, lemon, orange, grape, berry, chocolate raspberry, root beer, English toffee, vanilla, cinnamon, peppermint, and hazelnut!

If you need to prepare a crust, try exchanging white flour for coarsely ground almonds, pecans, or walnuts (or you can use a combination of almond flour and cold pressed olive oil — your choice).

Sugar

Since I tear this non-nutrient to pieces in Chapter 11, I make do now by simply saying it's bad for you in so many ways. Worse yet, you don't always know you're eating it. Table 17-1 highlights the many disguises that sugar uses in food labels.

Table 17-1	The Many Names of Sugar	
Basic Sugars	*Syrups*	*The "ose" Sugar Names*
Brown (dark or light)	Corn	Dextrose
Coarse	Fructose or high fructose	Fructose
Confectioner's	Maple	Glucose
Liquid	Molasses	Lactose
Raw	Rice	Maltose
Sanding	Sorghum	Sucrose (saccharose)
White sugar (fine, extra fine, and granulated)		Xylose

Sugar and type 2 diabetes

More than any other disease, I find that type 2 diabetes has the biggest collection of myths and old wives' tales surrounding it. Upwards of 300 million people worldwide suffer from this type of diabetes. Type 2 diabetes is not something you're born with, it's a disease that develops when your body can no longer make or use insulin. *Insulin* is a hormone that regulates your blood sugar; your pancreas controls the insulin release when sugar enters your blood stream. Eat a bag of candy? Your pancreas releases insulin. Like little soldiers — the insulin marches into your bloodstream to clean up the mess of sugar there.

It's believed that after years of blood sugar spikes (resulting from ingesting too much sugar over and over) the body becomes *insulin resistant* meaning that your insulin hormones are no longer effective at combating the sugar in the blood. This situation can take years to diagnose, as the outward symptoms of type 2 diabetes are not as readily apparent as those of someone who is born diabetic (type 1 diabetes). However, type 2 diabetes can be dangerous and may lead to heart disease, insulin dependence, circulation problems (especially in the feet), skin changes, and vision problems. Think about this the next time you choose a fountain soda size — a 44-ounce non-diet soda can average more than 100 grams of sugar (or a little over three-quarters of a cup), depending on the brand. Can you imagine sitting down and eating three-quarters of a cup of sugar?

Consider exchanging the acidifying sugars for:

✔ Stevia

✔ Honey (in moderation — this one's pH effect on the body is under debate)

✔ Natural fruit sweetness

Dairy

Heavy cream, butter, and ice cream make many a delightful dessert dish — but they all stem from one product: milk. Although milk is full of protein and vitamin D, it's also an animal product that acidifies your tissues. In most baked goods, the dairy takes on two roles: a source of fat (butter) and a source of moisture (milk or cream).

Although it will probably take some experimenting, consider exchanging common dairy ingredients for:

- ✔ Unsweetened applesauce
- ✔ Ripe, mashed bananas
- ✔ Almond or soy milk
- ✔ Clarified butter (which is butter with the milk fats removed; see the recipe in Chapter 13)
- ✔ Soy or no-fat yogurt

Eggs

At the ripe age of five, my oldest son saw me whipping eggs into cake batter and decided he would never eat a cake again (he's an egg-hater). Eggs have a couple functions in traditional dessert recipes. They help to *leaven* the dish (make it fluffy) and keep the ingredients stuck together, acting as a cohesive agent. In most dessert recipes, you can substitute egg whites without altering the end result too much. Egg replacement products are a little trickier to use, as most of them come in a powdered form and don't work too well as a leavening agent.

Creating a Balanced Dessert

I chose these dessert recipes with simplicity in mind. If you are a gourmet cook or a baker, you can experiment with your own recipes, remembering the aforementioned exchanges. I like these recipes because I can pronounce every ingredient on the list and don't have to drive across town to find outrageous items included in some of the alkaline dessert recipes I've seen (really, where do you find flaxseed gel?). The ingredients I selected have minimal pH impact and won't add cups of acid to your system — unlike the majority of store-bought goodies.

Silky Lemon Pie

Ditch the box of processed lemon pie mix, which probably contains acidifying sugars, gelatins, and other fillers. You can make your own filling using silken tofu and real lemons (wow!). If you don't want to take the time to make your own pie crust, treat the filling like a thick pudding — spoon it into a bowl, then into your mouth.

You may be unfamiliar with soy and psyllium powders, which I use in this recipe. In the filling, the soy powder provides a little protein boost (hey, desserts can be nutritious). In the crust, the psyllium powder helps bind the ingredients together and it provides a little extra fiber to keep your digestive tract happy!

Prep time: 15 minutes • **Cook time:** 10 minutes • **Yield:** 4 to 6 servings

Lemon Pie Filling

12 ounces silken tofu, drained **Juice of 1 lemon**	**1** In a blender, mix the tofu, lemon juice, ½ tablespoon lemon zest, and stevia thoroughly.
1½ tablespoons lemon zest, divided **2 tablespoons soy powder, optional**	**2** Slowly sprinkle in the soy powder, if desired, and blend for 1 more minute.
2 1-gram Stevia packets, or ½ teaspoon stevia powder, or 8 drops liquid, or 1 teaspoon minced leaves	

Pie Crust

1 cup almonds, soaked overnight	**1** Slip the almonds from their skins and discard the skins.
½ cup dates **½ tablespoon cold-pressed olive oil**	**2** Place the almonds, dates, olive oil, psyllium powder, and remaining lemon zest in a food processor. Mix until thoroughly blended.
1 teaspoon psyllium powder	**3** Firmly press the almond mixture into the pie dish, evenly coating the bottom and sides. Add 1 tablespoon of water if the mixture is too dry to press into the pie dish.

Putting it together

1 Pour Lemon Pie Filling into homemade Pie Crust, and refrigerate for at least 2 hours before serving.

Per serving: Calories 338 (From Fat 202); Fat 22g (Saturated 2g); Cholesterol 0mg; Sodium 16mg; Carbohydrate 28g; Dietary Fiber 6g; Protein 13g.

Better Baked Apples

Don't toss those overly ripe apples — slice and bake them to surprise your family with a healthy dessert after dinner tonight. If the aroma of roasting apples isn't enough to have them running to the kitchen, try serving the apples with an almond-based, dairy-free ice cream substitute, which you can find in the freezer section of most health food stores.

Prep time: 15 minutes • **Cook time:** 45 minutes • **Yield:** 6 servings

Ingredients	*Directions*
6 small apples, cored and thickly sliced	*1* Preheat the oven to 350 degrees. Grease a baking pan with a dash of the clarified butter, and line the bottom with the sliced apples.
1 and ½ tablespoons cinnamon, divided	
3 1-gram packets Stevia, or ¾ teaspoon powder, or 12 drops liquid, or 2 teaspoons fresh minced leaves, divided	*2* Mix 1 tablespoon of cinnamon and 2 packets of stevia in a small bowl; sprinkle this mixture over the apples.
½ cup almond flour	*3* Hand whip the almond flour, remaining stevia, and cinnamon, water, and egg white until mixed. Pinch off little pieces of the doughy mix and drop them over the apples.
¼ cup water	
1 egg white, or substitute equivalent	*4* Drizzle clarified butter over the top of the dish, and bake for about 45 minutes.
⅓ cup clarified butter	

Per serving: Calories 222 (From Fat 147); Fat 16g (Saturated 7g); Cholesterol 29mg; Sodium 13mg; Carbohydrate 18g; Dietary Fiber 5g; Protein 3g.

Note: I like to use a 9-x-9 pan for this dish. You can peel the apples if you find the dessert is too bitter, but I like the fiber in the peels.

Fast cocoa facts

Contrary to some outrageous claims I've heard, you *can* eat cocoa on an acid alkaline diet. The most alkalinizing choice is raw organic cocoa — not the creamy concoctions lining the check out aisle (those are stuffed with milk and sugars, which negatively impact your pH). Studies show that cocoa in moderation is good for your health and wellbeing because:

✔ It decreases inflammation throughout the body (decreasing risk of heart attack and stroke).

✔ Cocoa stimulates *endorphin* (*happy chemical*) release and can combat stress.

✔ It is a plant food full of *antioxidants*, which are substances that neutralize pollution in your body (cellular waste, infection, and inflammation).

Just don't make a meal out of chocolate. Scientists say about 6 or 7 grams a day will do the trick for your health — or less than an ounce of cocoa a day.

Oatmeal Cookies

These will be gone as fast as you can bake them. Watch out for the stampede as would-be cookie-eaters run to the kitchen to claim these while they're hot. Rolled oats are one of the few non-acidifying grains, and they make one heck of a cookie.

Prep time: 10 minutes • **Cook Time:** 15 minutes • **Yield:** 14 to 16 servings

Ingredients	Directions
2 cups rolled oats	**1** Preheat the oven to 350 degrees. In a large bowl, mix together the oats, almond flour, salt, stevia, baking powder, and baking soda. Set aside.
1 cup almond flour	
¼ teaspoon salt	
12 1-gram Stevia packets, or 3 teaspoons stevia powder, or 14 drops liquid, or 6 teaspoons minced fresh leaves	**2** In a small bowl, mix together the butter, vanilla, almond milk, and egg whites.
½ teaspoon baking powder	**3** Pour the butter mixture into the dry ingredients and mix thoroughly. Add mashed banana and mix.
½ teaspoon baking soda	
½ cup clarified butter	**4** Scoop mix by rounded tablespoon onto baking sheet and cook for 15 minutes.
Dash of vanilla extract (alcohol free)	
1 tablespoon almond milk	
2 egg whites, or ½ cup prepared egg substitute	
1 ripe banana, mashed	

Per serving: Calories 164 (From Fat 109); Fat 12g (Saturated 5g); Cholesterol 19mg; Sodium 112mg; Carbohydrate 10g; Dietary Fiber 4g; Protein 4g.

Note: The banana replaces the shortening or lard in traditional oatmeal cookie recipes.

Banana Bars

Satisfy your sweet tooth while getting your fiber and potassium in one yummy rectangle of goodness. If you're ready to start experimenting, you can nix the lemon zest and stevia powder and add a couple drops of your favorite flavored liquid stevia blend (think orange or apricot!) instead.

Prep time: 10 minutes • **Cook time:** 20 minutes • **Yield:** 8 to 10 servings

Ingredients	Directions
1 teaspoon clarified butter	*1* Preheat the oven to 275 degrees. Line a baking sheet with parchment paper and grease the paper with butter.
1 ½ cups rolled oats	
1 ripe banana	
¾ cup ground almonds	*2* Place the oats, banana, almonds, stevia, and lemon zest in a food processor and mix well.
1-gram packet Stevia, or ¼ teaspoon powder, or ½ teaspoon fresh minced leaves	
1 teaspoon lemon zest	*3* Pour oat mixture onto the baking sheet and spread it evenly, pressing it flat.
	4 Bake for 15 to 20 minutes, or until desired crispness achieved. Cool before cutting into bars.

Per serving: Calories 127 (From Fat 55); Fat 6g (Saturated 1g); Cholesterol 1mg; Sodium 1mg; Carbohydrate 15g; Dietary Fiber 3g; Protein 5g.

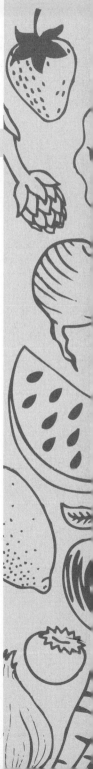

Fruit Kabobs

What could be easier than sticking a bunch of fruit on a stick and tossing it on the grill? Grilling fruit for dessert is almost that easy. Some fruits don't grill well (think watermelon), but the majority of them taste even better lightly cooked. Grilling brings out the natural sweetness, which alleviates the need for any sticky or whipped toppings that aren't so good pH-wise.

Soak fruit before grilling to have a moist treat. To get your fruit ready for the grill:

- ✔ Wash and dry the fruit thoroughly. Keep peels on the fruit and slice or halve the fruits.

- ✔ Place fruit in a large bowl filled with water. Add 1 tablespoon lemon juice per 2 cups of water to keep fruits from browning. Soak for about 30 minutes.

Try not to wander too far from the grill while dessert is on, or you may end up with a caramelized blob of mush.

Cooking time varies on how you like your fruit — I like it just barely caramelized, which takes just under 10 minutes. (Too much longer than that and the structure of the fruit starts to break down.)

Prep time: 30 minutes • **Cook time:** 10 minutes • **Yield:** 6 to 8 servings

Ingredients	*Directions*
Half a pineapple	*1* Lightly oil a clean, cold, outdoor grill.
4 bananas	
Honeydew melon	*2* Thoroughly wash and dry all fruits.
2 oranges	*3* Remove the stem from the pineapple, cut it in half, and core the half you're going to use. Slice the pineapple into 1-inch slices, leaving the outer skin intact.
Lemon juice	
Water	
	4 Slice the bananas in half lengthwise, and keep the skin intact.
	5 Cut the honeydew melon in half, seed it, then cut each half in quarters. Repeat until 1 inch slices remain, leaving outer skin intact.

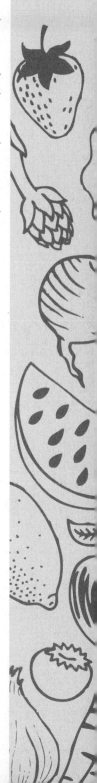

6 Quarter the oranges and remove seeds. Leave the peels intact.

7 In a large bowl, cover fruits with water and add lemon juice as needed to retain coloring. Soak for about 30 minutes.

8 Preheat the grill to medium low. Arrange fruit on the grill with skins initially facing down. Grill for 6 to 8 minutes per side.

9 Take the fruit off the grill. Chop the bananas, melon, and pineapple into 2-inch pieces. Place the fruits on wooden skewers for presentation.

Per serving: *Calories 209 (From Fat 9); Fat 1g (Saturated 0g); Cholesterol 0mg; Sodium 19mg; Carbohydrate 54g; Dietary Fiber 6g; Protein 2g.*

Part V
Overcoming Obstacles to Your pH Goals

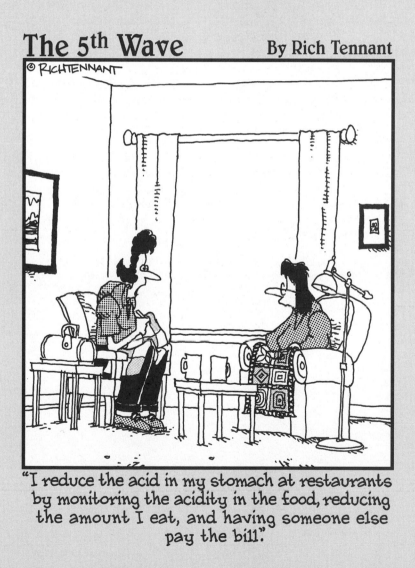

The 5th Wave   By Rich Tennant

"I reduce the acid in my stomach at restaurants by monitoring the acidity in the food, reducing the amount I eat, and having someone else pay the bill."

In this part...

1 cover all of those conundrums that usually get people off track in a pH balanced diet. Guess what? You can still eat out at your favorite restaurant and take the cake at a birthday party. I'm a big fan of living — really living — and I wouldn't adhere to any diet that disallowed it.

The acid alkaline diet promotes a balance of fresh veggies, fruits, and healthy proteins. Whatever else you put in your mouth is going to impact your pH, but these chapters show you how to work around acid-forming favorites, holiday staples, and even reach out for support when you need a little extra help.

I wrap it up by helping you discover (and avoid) common weight loss mistakes. Although the acid alkaline diet isn't intended solely for dropping pounds, it's a pretty nice side effect of a healthy diet.

Chapter 18

Dining Out

• •

In This Chapter

▶ Deciding on a cuisine

▶ Ordering pH-friendly fare

▶ Ordering to suit your diet and yourself

▶ Enjoying the occasional social engagement

▶ Avoiding pH conundrums

• •

While you're working hard to balance your pH and strive for a healthier lifestyle, life as you know it continues. Your kids still want to go to the Friday night pizza buffet, and friends from work are hosting a party at the new chophouse down the road. One of the best things about the acid alkaline diet is its versatility — you don't have to count carbs, calories, or log every morsel that enters your mouth. As long as you have a grasp of what foods to embrace and which ones to avoid, you're on the right track.

Restaurateurs are not simple people — they are savvy businessmen and women who know how to dress up a menu and make your mouth water. They also know that the majority of people prefer their veggies camouflaged and their meat overwhelming the plate (hence the 28-ounce prime rib I saw on a menu the other night — honestly, who needs that much meat?). This chapter helps you break the restaurant menu code; you can leave any establishment with your pH intact by doing your homework and employing savvy ordering techniques.

Choosing the Establishment

If you have a vote, certain restaurants are more pH friendly than others. I work pretty hard for my paycheck so I can't name names (and suffer a massive lawsuit), but I can illustrate which establishments offer more alkaline foods and less acidifying choices.

Selecting your dining style

Eating establishments are categorized not only by price and fare, but also by their service type. The basic types include:

- ✔ **Gourmet:** Elegant and usually pricey, gourmet restaurants are usually considered four- or five-star establishments. Professional chefs prepare your meal, and each menu item is freshly prepared, cooked on site (not just reheated), and artfully presented. The menu choices may be limited depending on the chef's preference, and unless you're a foodie, you may not recognize some of the fancier dishes.

- ✔ **Family/casual dining:** These establishments usually host a large, standardized menu and may be personally owned or part of a larger franchise. These family- and child-friendly establishments can usually accommodate food exchanges upon request (broccoli instead of white potatoes, for example).

- ✔ **Fast casual:** Found everywhere nowadays, these are homogenized versions of fast food and casual dining. You sit down and get served a meal, but the menu selections are not much better than most fast food joints.

- ✔ **Fast food:** Just like the name implies, you walk or drive up, order your food, and are eating it within minutes. The menu items are limited and are mostly relegated to the world of fried foods, burgers, and tacos.

Without pinpointing specific restaurant chains, you're probably going to find the best option for a healthy, alkaline meal at a family/casual or gourmet restaurant. The food costs a little more, but the servers are usually willing to take specific cooking instructions and swap out acid-forming sides (think French fries) for healthier, more alkaline-forming side dishes (steamed broccoli).

Enjoying international cuisine

When I eat out, I like to enjoy a dish that I can't (or don't know how to) make at home. But I have to be choosy in my cuisine selection, because some types of international cuisine are more pH friendly than others:

- ✔ **American** cuisine reflects its melting pot of ancestry and is usually colored by geographical location. Dishes range from barbequed meats to deep dish pizzas and everything in between. Wheat, dairy, beef, and fried foods are staples in most American diets, which is why they've gained the nickname of the Standard American Diet, or *SAD* for short.

Your best bet in American fare is to eat a large salad (olive oil for dressing) and request steamed veggies instead of fries, mashed potatoes, or any number of the other starches usually offered. The least acidic choices may include a steamed seafood dish in the northeast or *naked* poultry (without breading) in the South.

✔ **Chinese** food is frequently offered in a buffet type of setting, where you can go haywire with calories, fried foods, and pounds of rice. If you have a hankering for it, fill up on the vegetable and egg-based soups before you hit the rest of the buffet. Leave the white rice — so acid-forming — to someone else and fill your plate with steamed veggies (broccoli) and a healthy protein like sautéed chicken or tofu.

✔ **Greek** and **Mediterranean** cuisine offer much in the way of alkalinizing fruits and vegetables. Mediterranean fare offers healthy choices such as the chicken shish kebab, which usually includes a mix of grilled peppers and other vegetables. Ask for wild rice on the side as opposed to the white rice or soft breads that usually accompany these dishes.

If you're going Greek, avoid the hummus and cheese pastries, both of which are acid-forming. Instead, elect to have grilled chicken or boiled shrimp. If you're adventurous, try a zucchini blossom stuffed with bulgur (the gorgeous orange flowers are very tasty and nicely alkaline-forming!).

Limit your dipping, because most of the condiments in Greek fare are yogurt-based. And if you want to enjoy a *dolmathakia* (stuffed grape leaves) — and who doesn't? — just remember to do so in moderation and pair it with plenty of alkaline-forming veggies.

✔ **Italian** cuisine gets tricky with the breading (think veal parmesan), pasta, and savory breads offered at most restaurants. If you want pasta, just remember that it's acid-forming (I doubt most restaurants carry spelt pasta), not to mention that many fine Italian restaurants deliver a single entrée containing multiple servings of pasta. However, some places are now carrying farro, which is a cousin to spelt. If they have this type of pasta, choose it without guilt.

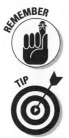

Keep proper serving sizes in mind. Just because you're served a mountain of spaghetti doesn't mean you have to eat it. Ball your fist — that's about one serving of pasta and all you should consume if you do indulge.

To add some alkaline to your Italian meal, load up on the *pesto* (fresh basil and garlic with olive oil), tomatoes, and garlic. You can also request parmesan dishes without breading, which helps to cut some of the acidic ingredients.

✔ **Japanese** food screams sushi and seaweed — if you get selective, you can find a very alkaline-friendly meal in these restaurants. Seaweed is one of the most alkaline-forming foods you can eat (and it's not something I routinely have on hand at home, so it's a nice treat).

Avoid the *tempuras,* which are tasty but nothing more than fried food. Instead, reach for the *sashimi,* which is raw fish sushi without the sticky acidifying white rice wrapper. Many of the Japanese soups are fish or vegetable-based (think *Yosenabe*) and are a great way to start the meal.

Raw or undercooked fish may contain parasites and are not advised for anyone with an immune system deficiency or disorder. Most gourmet sushi chefs freeze the raw fish before serving it, which helps to kill parasites. (But better safe than sorry.)

- ✔ **Mexican** food can be enjoyed on the acid alkaline diet, but it takes some fancy footwork. The majority of dishes are corn-based (tamales, tortillas) and if you're not in Mexico City, they've also been Europeanized to some extent with loads of acid-forming cheese.

Stick to the fajitas, which are usually filled with a mixture of grilled veggies and meat. Select the chicken or shrimp fajitas and request steamed vegetables over the *frijoles refritos* (refried beans). Likewise, avoid the heaping servings of Spanish rice, which contain the acid-forming ingredients of yellow rice and corn. Instead, reach for dishes made with avocadoes, guava, peppers, and papaya.

- ✔ **Thai** and **Southeast Asian** foods are a very pH friendly choice if you avoid the fried and battered foods. Thai dishes usually incorporate a delicious marriage of spices and alkalinizing veggies like garlic and cabbage, and they offer a plethora of vegetarian, spicy fish, and chicken dishes.

Feel free to load up on the Thai dipping sauces, which are traditionally made of lime juice (very alkaline-forming), garlic, and chilies.

Grab a bowl of vegetable-based seaweed soup (*tom chuet taohu kap sarai*) if you're headed to a buffet. It's alkaline-forming, fills your belly, and it can extinguish the fire on your tongue after eating some of the traditional spicier dishes.

Weighing in at the food court

A study by the Center for Science in the Public Interest (CSPI) showed that if you get hit with hunger pangs in the mall and stop for a snack at the food court, the calorie-count of your snack may be much higher than you realize. Shopping center food courts are notoriously laden with calorie-engorged choices, most of which are quick and convenient to the shopper on a mission.

The worst part? Some of the food choices sound perfectly innocuous. When I stop for a slice of dripping-with-cheese pizza or a milkshake, I know I'm in for extra calories. But when I stop and grab a sub shop sandwich, it seems like I am making a better choice for my waistline . . . or am I? Try to match the food court selections in the lettered list with the calories in the numbered list. The numbers are from a report by the CSPI, "Food Courts: Fattening Americans as They Shop."

A. Coffee-chain mocha

B. Slice of mall pizza

C. Steak sub and French fries

D. Frozen yogurt with toppings

E. Large meat and cheese sandwich from a sandwich chain

1. 1,300 calories

2. 800 calories

3. 2,000 calories

4. 700 calories

5. 600 calories

Answers: A) 5, B) 2, C) 3, D) 4, E) 1

Bet you'll think twice the next time you feel like grabbing a quick meal between stores!

Everything in moderation

I'm sure the die-hard alkalarians gasp when they see me saying that you can eat (but limit) pasta, meats, and a wide variety of international fare when you dine out. I'm not saying it's okay to do daily, but there's nothing wrong with occasionally sampling all of life's bounty in moderation.

What a dull existence this would be if I could never sample an authentic tamale in Nogales or try a spoonful of homemade ice cream on a farm in North Carolina. My motto: Stay aware of pH, and eat the majority of selections from alkaline-forming foods, but don't miss out on life.

Making Food Selections

I applaud you if you're already ordering more vegetables and less meat, but take it a step further to make the meal truly alkaline-heavy. The magicians in the kitchen add sauces, toppings, and all kinds of flavorful ingredients that abracadabra your boring dish into something incredible. At the same time, they're usually making otherwise healthy dishes — think baked sweet potato — pH *un*friendly with the added ingredients (think baked sweet potato topped with butter, sugar, and marshmallows).

I wish I could contribute one entire page to this statement:

Foods listed as "light fare" or "healthy" do not always translate as good for your pH. For the most part, foods listed as "healthy" on a menu only need to have a reduced calorie content. Instead of eating a 1,200-calorie bowl of macaroni and cheese, the "healthy" version uses less butter and two percent milk, making you suffer only 600 calories. Sure, these items may be the lesser evil, but what you want to avoid is the acid-forming ingredients, not just the calories.

Simplifying salads

Ordering a salad seems like a perfectly alkaline choice, right? Yes, so long as it's not drowned in fatty dressing, croutons, bacon, cheese, and all the other acid-forming things available to add.

It takes time, but eventually your taste buds appreciate the natural flavors of a vegetable medley without an entire jar — or even a tablespoon — of dressing. Trust me on this one.

One of the worst pH offenders in the salad arena is the classic Caesar salad. Romaine lettuce leaves are thoroughly coated in a cream-based dressing and then piled with croutons and cheese. You may actually be better off eating those French fries as opposed to this monstrosity!

Pick a classic tossed or garden salad, and ask your server what comes on it. Ask him or her to keep these items off:

- Bacon or other meat
- Cheese
- Croutons
- Dressing
- Eggs

Instead of ranch, blue cheese, or Italian dressing, opt for olive oil and a teeny dash of vinegar (balsamics are acid-forming, so take it easy on the dash). But remember, one tablespoon of olive oil packs over 100 calories, so don't suffocate your greens in the stuff.

Navigating side dishes

On the acid alkaline diet, side dishes can make or break the meal. Most establishments offer a variety of vegetables, legumes, and starches for their sides. Even the healthy-sounding sides, like a broccoli casserole, can become a dish of acid with a little help from the kitchen staff. Ask your server how the veggie is prepared, if it comes with any toppings, and if they can put the toppings on the side.

Steer clear of the acid-forming starches, like white potatoes (in any form — mashed, baked, fried, scalloped) and corn. The other steamed veggies are pH- friendly as long as they're not smothered in oils, cheese, or butter sauce.

Engaging appetizers

Appetizers are those delicious morsels you eat before the meal. Usually rich and gooey (think loaded potato skins), they're particularly poor for your pH balance. Of course, the appetizers available vary depending on the cuisine you choose. Right off the bat I can think of at least three American appetizers that I wouldn't touch with a pitchfork:

- Fried vegetables or cheese
- Creamy dips and chips
- Loaded nachos or fries

Even if you want to forget about your pH for the next half-hour, consider your heart and waistline. Restaurant-style mozzarella sticks pack over 750 calories per serving and provide 44 whopping fat grams according to the U.S. Department of Agriculture, Agricultural Research Service.

If it's too difficult to resist (or you're starving), consider sharing a small appetizer around the table or picking a more alkaline-friendly fare. Shrimp cocktail, spring rolls, sushi, soup, or salad can take the edge off of your hunger pangs without dropping your pH too much.

While you're waiting on your steaming entrée, ask for a large glass of lemon water. Drink it before your meal, and I bet you eat less and feel better later.

Putting it all together with entrees

Each entrée is typically created around a protein. If you're unsure or don't know what proteins have the biggest pH impact, check the list I made for you in Chapter 11.

Proteins are not the stars in acid alkaline meals; the alkalinizing vegetables should take center stage.

While you're perusing the protein selections:

✔ Look for the words baked, broiled, or grilled

✔ Stick to a serving (that's about the size of a deck of cards) of protein

✔ Choose the least acid-forming entrees such as chicken or salmon

Placing Your Order

You are the customer. You get it the way you want it, or you eat somewhere else. Don't be afraid to ask questions and order your meal exactly the way you want it. Specifying how you want your food cooked can save you a lot of heartache while watching your pH. Any food can become acid-forming and tip your scales if you let it. Just imagine frying a piece of kale and dipping it in a creamy ranch dip. It used to be an alkalinizing dark green veggie, now it's breaded, fried, and smothered in acid-forming ingredients.

Picking your preparation method

The restaurant chef should be able to honor reasonable requests such as:

✔ Hold the sauce, butter, or creams

✔ Steam or grill the food as opposed to frying or sautéing in oils

✔ Use cooking spray instead of oil for grilled foods

✔ Alter portion sizes (double the veggie, halve the protein)

So you have a hankering for some chicken wings, do you? There's two things you can do to make this a less acid-forming choice — ask for them without breading and have them baked, not fried.

Watching the portions

Can you say, "portion overload?" It's always best to assume that you're going to get two or maybe even three servings of each food when you eat out.

On one hand it's good, because you want to get the most for your hard-earned money. However, you may be eating two or three extra servings of an acid-forming food if you do as mother said and clean your plate.

Ask for a to-go container as soon as your food is served. Cut your meal in half, and save it for tomorrow.

Eating out with a group

Whether it's a work or social event, you're probably going to dine with a group of co-workers or friends at some point. I have to attend many of these mandatory fun functions and always dread knowing I have a choice of tasteless fish or tasteless chicken awaiting me (the one I don't order always looks better).

It's perfectly acceptable to pass on any food that doesn't fit in your acid alkaline diet.

Because the group dining choices are usually relegated to the land of chicken, beef, or fish, I inquire about vegetarian substitutions in advance. Sure, I eat chicken every now and then, but if the restaurant can provide a healthier option, I'll take it! Just make sure that their idea of a vegetarian meal doesn't include a deep fried veggie or breaded eggplant. In that case, it may be safer for your pH to stick with chicken.

It probably started as "Caesar's salad"

Although stories are conflicting (and many people would like to take credit for the creation), there's a good chance that the Roman emperor did not enjoy this famous dish of greens nor was it actually named after him. As many believe to be the case, the first documented Caesar salad was probably served in Tijuana, Mexico, during the 1920's. Seeing as how Julius Caesar died in 44 B.C., that's about a 1,960-year discrepancy, give or take.

Many accounts credit the Italian-born chef, Caesar Cardini with the creation. A restaurant owner and chef, Cardini was credited with preparing his salad (quickly referred to as "Caesar's salad") at the tableside.

Unlike the store-bought bottled dressings seen in most restaurants today, the original Caesar salad grew infamous due to its creamy and unusual dressing made with almost raw egg yolks, garlic, and anchovies.

A century later, few people consume raw egg products anymore, no matter how delicious they made Caesar's salad. The fear of contracting *salmonella,* a dangerous bacterium that causes diarrhea and foodborne illness, is too great.

Doing Your Homework

Check out the menu before you get stuck at a certain restaurant. Ideally, the establishment has a website where you can check out their fare (and sometimes even the nutritional values) prior to committing. If you forget to check online, many establishments have a menu posted near the door, or you can request one from the maitre d'.

No one said you couldn't eat at a steakhouse anymore, just be aware that the majority of the menu items consist of beef. It's like going to a seafood restaurant when you have a craving for poultry — probably not the best choice for someone who is pH conscientious.

I like to find restaurants that have a smashing salad bar. They are few and far between — most establishments have a sad collection of wilted iceberg lettuce, cucumbers, chopped egg, stale croutons, and cheese. If you're lucky they have tomatoes that don't look anemic. Ask to check out the salad bar before you decide to eat there.

Finding the right answers

Aside from the rare establishment that posts nutrition values right up on their menu board, trying to find the nutrient data for some restaurants may feel a bit like pulling teeth. To get ingredient and nutrient data you can ask:

✔ Your waiter or waitress, the restaurant maitre d', manager, or owner.

✔ The opinion of your nutritionist, or you can see if he or she has any information (nutrition professionals have better access to such things).

✔ Online local chat board participants — someone may know what you want to know.

Many free calorie counters and smartphone apps provide a program for tracking restaurant nutrition. They're still limited to the most popular items, but at least they show the massive amounts of fat, sodium, and calories stuffed into many famous entrees.

Admitting weakness

Mine would be a piping-hot deep-dish pizza. It takes zero effort to realize that I cannot enter an establishment that offers the best pizza in town without succumbing to a slice (or two or three). So, what do I do? I don't go there. I've been saying moderation is key and illustrating how to eat out while still keeping it alkaline, but now I'm adding a caveat: Avoid your old acid-forming stomping grounds.

If the magnetic pull towards a certain acid-forming food is too much to tolerate, don't make yourself suffer by watching other people eat it.

Embracing the Social Toast

Toasting is a time-honored practice carried out in almost every region (excluding Muslim societies, where alcohol is forbidden). It's used to honor special guests and break the ice during social events. The small sips of wine or other alcohol ingested during a toast is probably not going to have a large impact on your pH. However, if you prefer not to drink, there are plenty of ways to fake it during a toast. Consider:

✔ Toasting with seltzer water with a slice of lemon or lime

✔ Raising your water glass

✔ Pretending to take tiny sips of the alcohol after each toast (your glass won't get refreshed between toasts that way)

Whatever beverage you choose to toast with, don't forget to add the most common words, "Cheers!" or "To your health!" before you raise the glass.

Common alcohol myths

Even if I didn't already know them from college, I've heard a scary number of alcohol untruths shared by inebriated would-be drivers. The fact is, if you plan to drink — no matter how little — plan on getting a ride home. A large study by the National Highway Traffic Safety Administration used the measurement of blood alcohol concentration (BAC) to test impaired responses in the average driver. It showed that alcohol could impair your ability to multi-task at BAC levels as low as 0.005 and your ability to judge lanes and traffic lines as low as 0.0018. The legal intoxication level varies by country, but in the United States and Canada, a BAC of 0.08 is considered legally intoxicated. Consider these myths the next time you think you may be safe to drive home:

✔ You won't get drunk if you have a full stomach. **False** — the alcohol will be absorbed more slowly, but you still suffer its intoxicating effects.

✔ Drink a glass of water after every alcoholic drink to avoid inebriation. **False** — water does help to keep you hydrated, but it's your liver that clears alcohol from your system and there's no known way to speed that process up.

✔ I've developed a tolerance and I can drink more than you without getting drunk. **False** — your blood alcohol content depends on your gender, body weight, and how fast you kick back the drinks.

Consuming wisely

Every type of alcohol is going to negatively impact your pH. I get this question a lot when people ask what type of alcohol is the best for you. There are no alkaline-forming alcohols out there. The high sugar content and fermentation process makes all alcohol acid-forming during digestion.

Studies are ongoing, but research suggests that a little (and I mean little) red wine may be the best choice for your heart and cardiovascular system. The evidence that people who consume red wine may have healthier hearts is lovingly nicknamed the French paradox, as the wine seems to offset the effects of the traditionally rich French diet.

But this heart-protecting benefit is tricky, and it's not foolproof. Worse yet, drinking alcohol can actually increase your risk of certain cancers, including those of the breast and the colon.

If you're going to consume, keep it safe and stop after one serving.

Making better choices

I don't want to offend, but I do want to put this out there: If the thought of giving up alcohol for your body's pH balance is enough to scare you away, you may want to consider asking for help. Alcoholism is a nasty, insidious disease that is sometimes very difficult to recognize and treat by yourself. There's no shame in asking for help to quit drinking if you need it.

Going to pubs with friends or sitting around a bonfire requires alcohol, right? Wrong. There are plenty of delicious, pH-friendly beverages that can take the place of an alcoholic one. The next time you're offered a glass of wine or beer consider drinking:

- ✔ A soda water with lemon, lime, or a splash of 100 percent cranberry juice
- ✔ Fresh squeezed fruit juice in sparkling water
- ✔ A frosty glass of mineral water

Navigating the Biggest pH Offenders

Some people mistakenly believe that you can only enjoy an alkalinizing diet at home by eating massive amounts of fruits and vegetables. This is not even close to accurate. As long as you steer clear of the top acid-forming foods and pile the alkaline-forming foods high on your plate, you can most certainly enjoy going out to eat occasionally.

Buffets don't kill your pH, you do

Here's a myth: Buffets make you fat and cannot be enjoyed on an acid alkaline diet. In my experience, I'm the only one that decides what goes into my mouth. The restaurant owners are not responsible for your pH, cardiac health, or your waistline.

You can control yourself at a buffet by remembering these tips:

- ✔ Fill up with a soup (non-cream based) or salad first.
- ✔ Avoid the fried island — look for the baked dishes and veggies.
- ✔ Just because the dessert's there doesn't mean you have to indulge.
- ✔ Unless this is your last meal, you do not have to eat your money's worth.
- ✔ Fill at least a quarter of your plate with fresh vegetables from the salad area.

Ask your server what else is available. I recently went to a Japanese-style buffet where I was able to order specialty items off a menu at no extra charge (of course I got the seaweed and sushi).

Dealing with fast food in a fast society

If you must, you can navigate fast food menus in a pinch (but I don't advise it). Many franchises have jumped on the healthy train and offer non-breaded cousins of their famous entrée or fruit slices and salads as a side item. If you have to eat fast food, look for these magic words on the menu: grilled or broiled.

If a salad is offered, make sure that the dressing and croutons come on the side (or pick them off). To make your choices less acid-forming you can also consider:

- Leaving off the condiments
- Ordering a bottle of water, not soda
- Choosing only small sizes
- Picking a wrap over a bun (or just tossing the bun)
- Skipping the sides unless fruit or veggie sticks are an option

Then go home and drink a big glass of lemon water (not kidding). Flush the remaining acids out of your system by making dinner from fresh, wholesome ingredients and watching your acid-forming intake for the next few days.

Chapter 19

Navigating Holidays and Special Occasions

··

··

*W*hen I think of reasons I've quit diets past, I usually place the blame squarely on holidays and special occasions (and if that doesn't work, I blame coworkers with donuts). The majority of foods we convene around are usually acid-forming decadent finger foods, mounds of roasted meats, and sweet confections of comfort. Special occasions present a challenge to any dieter, but it's not insurmountable. This chapter helps you understand how to make better choices for your pH while deploying sly etiquette skills.

I like to stress the point that the acid alkaline diet is not aimed towards weight loss, it's geared towards a healthy, pH balanced body. If you fall off the pH wagon you can get right back on. Although I cover the basics of how to enjoy yourself and still stick to an alkaline-forming diet, how often you cheat on your journey to health is up to you.

Enjoying Big Food Holidays

Regardless of your culture, many religious and national holidays center on food. I can think of infamous offenders such as Thanksgiving — a big turkey-eating day in Canada and the United States — and religious holidays like Christmas or Hanukkah. One beautiful aspect of the acid alkaline diet is the fact that you can still partake in traditional foods during a holiday without all the guilt that calorie counters and carb cutters suffer. You just have to understand how to combat their acid-forming potential.

Holidays around the world

Holidays break down into three different types: the religious-based days, the national or country-affiliated celebrations, and holidays based in tradition. The religious-based holidays are more globally recognized due to the migration of people across continents, whereas the national and traditional holidays are usually only celebrated by certain cultural groups.

Holidays and holiday foods also correspond to the seasons:

✔ **Springtime** offerings include a variety of citrus foods, leafy greens, berries, asparagus, and artichoke. Some of the holidays celebrated in this season include Easter, Passover, May Day, Cinco de Mayo (fifth of May), and Walpurgisnacht (a Halloween-like European holiday).

✔ **Summer** harvest debuts with peaches, nectarines, and all varieties of peppers. As the season progresses, you can find watermelons, grapes, tomatoes, and eggplants fresh at the market. Independence Day is celebrated in the United States during the peak of summer. For Muslims throughout the world, the end of summer brings Ramadan, which is followed by the feast Id-Ul-Fitr.

✔ **Autumn** provides apples, pears, and corn early in the season. Pumpkins and squash, nuts and olives mature and are canned or stored for the remaining year. Rosh Hashanah, Yom Kippur, and Halloween are celebrated in many different countries during autumn. Mexico enjoys a three-day feast to respect the deceased called *El Día de los Muertos* (day of the dead).

✔ **Winter** is a time of rest for many farmers, although you can still find fresh beets and other root vegetables including carrots in the winter. Fresh broccoli, cauliflower, and collards are usually available throughout the season. Winter is bursting with food-rich holidays including Christmas, Hanukkah, Kwanzaa, New Year's Day, Chinese New Year, and Mardi Gras.

Every day is not a holiday or special occasion (well, for most of us). I am a huge advocate of living life to its fullest — don't walk away from that platter of latkes because they won't fit into your acid alkaline diet! Instead, learn how to pile alkaline-forming foods on your plate to combat the occasional acid-forming one.

Embracing seasonal advantages

Thank goodness for cold storage and warm regions — otherwise I couldn't enjoy my favorite fruits and vegetables year round. Our ancestors didn't have that luxury. They had to wait until the end of summer to enjoy a thick slice of watermelon or until autumn for pumpkins and apples.

That is how many of our holiday food traditions began — our ancestors were able to enjoy different grains, vegetables, and fruits at a specific time due to the changing seasons and harvest. These foods were then incorporated into the season's holidays. I've never heard of eating pumpkin pie for Passover or Easter, have you?

Use the seasons to your advantage. Many alkaline-forming foods are only available for a short time in their freshest, non-canned state. If you're an iceberg-lettuce-is-the-only-vegetable-I-eat kind of person, consider expanding your alkaline potential by adding these foods to your seasonal holiday spread:

- ✔ Plums, peaches, strawberries, and bell peppers in the summer
- ✔ Citrus, leafy greens (such as endive), and asparagus in the spring
- ✔ Apples, pumpkin seeds, and cinnamon in the fall
- ✔ Sweet potatoes, beets, broccoli, and cabbage in the winter

Striking a balance

Be conscious of your plate and portion sizes as you enjoy holiday goodies. I like to call it "looking at the big picture." If a special food linked to the holiday is acid-forming, as many of the meat and dough concoctions are, consider how you can arrange alkaline-forming foods on your plate to compensate for that indulgence.

If you've ever taken part in a Christmas feast, you already know what a plate full of acid-forming food looks like. Huge roasts, stuffing, fresh duck, and even a ham can decorate just one table. The side dishes may include buttery mashed potatoes, cranberries, and several types of pie.

You need to balance your acid and alkaline-forming holiday foods and beverages. Look at the whole day of food — the appetizers and finger foods, the entrée and side dishes, the beverages, and the desserts. A plate of lamb, roasted potatoes, baklava, and milk has no alkaline-forming buffers — it's *all* acidifying. A more pH-friendly version would include a small serving of lamb paired with a glass of lemon water and some roasted asparagus or peppers. Exchange the dessert for some seasonal fruits (or have a tiny piece of your traditional one) and you have an alkaline-forming holiday meal without having to sit in a corner eating tofu.

Recalling the 80/20 rule

I talk a lot about the 80/20 and the 60/40 rules in Chapter 2. If you're trying to restore your health, eating 80 percent alkaline-forming foods and only 20 percent acid-forming foods (per meal) is the way to go. If you're trying to maintain health or just want a more liberal approach to the acid alkaline diet, you can use the modified version of that: 60 percent alkaline-forming foods and 40 percent acid-forming ones.

Picking an acid and sticking with it

Another holiday option is to pick your most desired traditional food and eat it — but make that your main acid-forming choice and stick to one serving. It's a trick I've employed often while on very strict diets, which the acid alkaline diet is not. I find that the more you deny yourself, the more you want to cheat or stop the diet altogether. So if you want a plum-filled pierogie for dessert — it's okay!

Don't be shy, ask

Some holiday dishes are obviously acid-forming (think *loukoumades* — deep-fried pastry puffs dipped in sugar). Others, like a delicious fruit salad, may seem innocuous until you learn that your neighbor mixes the fruit in a dressing of sugar and mayonnaise.

You can't always tell what's in a dish just by eyeballing it — so go ahead and ask. Acid-forming ingredients are sneaky — you don't know what's in Aunt Hilda's famous wild rice casserole unless you ask her. Chances are, she'll be flattered you inquired, and you'll know whether or not to avoid (or limit) it on your plate.

Digging into Special Occasions

Weddings, birthday parties, and other special occasions don't always provide much time for you to plan ahead and alkalinize your body. Although simply avoiding the buffet table or the gigantic cake is an option, it probably won't be feasible for long. Eventually people may wonder why you never eat (is she a vampire?), and eventually you'll get sick of abstaining. Never fear, you have a couple ways to make pH-friendly decisions during these events and still remain in the social fray of things.

That cup of eggnog is costly

The creamy blend of eggnog is probably one of the worst (if not the worst) holiday drinks you can enjoy. One cup packs over 300 calories and more fat than most people eat in a whole day. Although the recipe is dependent on your geographical location, most eggnog blends contain eggs, sugar, whole milk, cream, nutmeg, vanilla, and a dash of rum, bourbon, or brandy. Apart from the nutmeg, pretty much everything in this drink is calorie-dense and acid-forming.

You have a number of options to make eggnog more pH-friendly:

✔ Have an eggnog *shot.* Pour yourself one or two ounces of the drink and sip slowly —

don't grab an eight-ounce glass and guzzle it. That's like mainlining cholesterol.

✔ Pull out the blender (or shaker) and mix ½ cup of the eggnog blend with ½ cup water, soymilk, or crushed ice to create a slightly diluted (in calories and acid) version of the drink you love.

✔ Make your own vegetarian eggnog using a mixture of silken tofu, soy or almond milk, stevia, vanilla, and nutmeg.

✔ Splurge during the holidays and purchase the pre-made soy or rice nogs in the dairy section at the grocery store. Sprinkle some nutmeg on top and enjoy.

Announcing "I'm a vegetarian"

Whether you're flying to Uncle Leo's birthday party or going to your brother's wedding, you can pull out the vegetarian card (figurative not literal). Most establishments and airlines have special vegetarian fare for people who don't eat meat. The special meal is less likely to be acid-forming than the traditional beef or chicken choice — as long as it's not breaded and fried. Ask what the vegetarian option is and then make your decision. If they smothered the fresh veggies in breading or oil, you may actually be better off selecting the chicken and eating a small (four ounce) serving.

Bringing your own dish

I've been to many parties where trays laden with cheese and roasted meats take center stage — I either ate the acid-forming foods and felt horrible later or I left hungry.

Don't assume that your host will provide healthy options. By bringing your own dish to share, you ensure that alkaline-forming foods are available.

You can make one of the salads or a crock-pot of soup mentioned in Chapter 14, or for something more informal, bring one of the many snacks I provide recipes for in Chapter 16. When all else fails, stop by the grocery store and pick up a fresh veggie tray and a loaf of sprouted bread on the way.

Examining your best pH choices

Striving to eat only healthy, alkalinizing food choices can be difficult when a small country's worth of food is set before you. It's not always easy to spot the healthy dish, but you can try adhering to these guidelines during an event:

- ✔ Avoid any dish covered in a heavy cream, gravy, or sauce.
- ✔ Use dips sparingly.
- ✔ Eat a large salad (alkaline-forming veggies) before you dig into the rest of the buffet or meal.
- ✔ Opt for small portions (four ounces or less) of salmon or skinless poultry as opposed to red meat or pork.
- ✔ Share the dessert or cake with someone or abstain altogether.

Vacations are good for you

Cheesy clichés aside (all work and no play), taking a vacation is a good way to restore mental health. Multiple research studies have concluded that people who take vacations from work have lower blood pressure and less stress hormones than the rest of us.

Whether your paradise of choice is a ski slope or a balmy beach, you need to recharge your mental batteries by taking some time off. Stress and getting inadequate rest are acid-forming. I bet if the researchers also checked urine pH during those studies, the vacationers would be far more alkaline than the people who didn't take time off.

If you don't have the financial reserves for your dream trip, consider taking a few days off (guilt-free) and do some local things you enjoy. You can put your mind into a vacation-like state by:

✔ Putting away all electronics on your time off. No smartphones, laptops, or anything else that tethers you to work and worries.

✔ Meditating, reading a book, or watching a good movie — they're ways to let your mind focus on something pleasant.

✔ Getting a massage. Massages not only release physical tension, there is emerging research that they also boost your brain's release of "happy" chemicals and can help ward off depression.

✔ Trying to get at least six to eight hours of uninterrupted sleep each night. Studies show that one of the biggest benefits of taking a vacation is that you sleep better — and longer — during and for a few days following the vacation.

Letting go on vacation

By definition, vacations are supposed to be a time of no stress — don't ruin that peaceful façade by obsessing over food choices. You can decrease the stress of the unknown restaurant menu by planning ahead and researching local establishments. Some other methods that help control vacation-induced acid splurges include:

✔ **Pack your own snacks,** especially if you're flying or driving. Kale chips, nuts, and seeds are easy to store. You can pack a cooler if you'd like to bring fresh vegetables, but some fruits, such as tangerines, do fine at room temperature for a day in the car.

✔ **Try a local alkaline-forming product** that you wouldn't typically make at home such as fresh sushi or produce from a farmer's stand.

✔ **Eat local fare and avoid the fast food** or commercialized restaurant chains if possible. Sit-down establishments have far more to offer in the way of healthy, alkaline-forming food choices than the fast food chains (even though many fast food chains are trying to get better at offering healthier choices).

Preparing to Party

Luckily for you, most special occasions and holidays have set dates — you know exactly when that upcoming event lands on your calendar. Take a look at your schedule and see what holidays, parties, or events are approaching and then plan your meals accordingly.

Loading up with alkaline

The week prior to an event, start loading up with alkaline-forming foods. Your pH will drop (become more acidic) when you eat acid-forming concoctions (wedding cake, cupcakes at that birthday party), but the insult to your body is less pronounced if you usually maintain an alkaline environment. It's like an Olympic athlete eating a slice of pizza — it's not the best food choice, but her body is in such phenomenal shape that it's not really going to matter in the long run (pun intended).

Eating before you go

It's not rude, it's smart. You know what foods you have stocked in your pantry at home, and you can control the portions of acid-forming foods you eat.

I like to eat a healthy meal of mostly green foods before I go to an event because then I'm not forced to eat whatever happens to be sitting on the buffet or served to me. At the very least, I like to grab an alkaline-forming snack, such as a glass of lemon water or a handful of pumpkin seeds, before I go to an event.

Balancing 24 hours

Your pH balance is constantly fluctuating according to what you eat, drink, and even how you're feeling. I discuss all the different things that influence pH in depth in Chapter 6, if you want to read more about that.

If you track urine or saliva pH, your measurements are going to drop and become slightly acidic for a while following a big food holiday or acid-forming food splurge. It's okay — this is your body's way of protecting you by getting rid of the acids. How long it takes to return to an alkaline state depends on your body and general health, how much you splurged, and what actions you take to correct the imbalance.

Repairing Celebratory Damage

Everyone makes bad food choices, some more frequently than others. The rate at which you recover from excessive acid intake depends on how fast your intestines process acid-forming foods and how quickly your liver and kidneys remove the acid.

What do you imagine would happen if you left the trash all over your house after a party? It would be unsanitary and eventually attract opportunistic rodents. Your body's no different. After you fill it with a special-occasion-induced acid overload, it's a good idea to clean house.

On your journey to a pH-balanced lifestyle, at some point, you may come across the term *potential renal acid load,* or PRAL for short. The fields of science and nutrition are researching how the PRAL measurements of food can predictably impact the acidity of your urine (technically called the *renal net acid excretion,* or NAE). Keep an eye out for breakthroughs — I'm a believer that science is going to keep exploring the acid alkaline diet until we know exactly how long it takes you to rid yourself of an acid-forming food. Current data is still not applicable to all of us because you may absorb and excrete minerals and protein faster than I do, or vice versa.

Loving your liver and kidneys

Together, your liver and kidneys are the crew ordained to clean up most biological messes in your body. They filter your blood and remove many acidifying substances including:

- ✔ Caffeine
- ✔ Fats
- ✔ Preservatives
- ✔ Tobacco and alcohol

Best practice is to avoid these substances on an acid alkaline diet, but even more so when you're trying to recover from a high level of acidity. When you eat foods or drinks containing these substances you actually increase the workload on your liver and kidneys, making it harder for them to do their job.

I'm not a proponent of detoxifying your liver and kidneys unless you do so with the guidance of a medical doctor. However, there are ways to improve their function and give them a little boost while they work to clear acids from your system. After a holiday or special-occasion acid splurge you can consider:

- Drinking plenty of fresh water.

- Loading up on supercharged greens such as spinach, kale, and broccoli.

- Eating more sprouted foods such as alfalfa.

- Drinking barley grass or dandelion tea, but only if your doctor gives approval. (Dandelion tea is not recommended for anyone with active gallbladder disease or stomach problems.)

- Enjoying some fresh watermelon — it's a natural diuretic.

- Getting out and exercising — exercise stimulates blood flow, which is vital to removing waste from your cells.

Stop harassing yourself

In most cases, you are your own worst enemy. It's human to think, "Well, I already wrecked my pH and went off the diet for the vacation, why should I go back on it?" This is a moment when it's important to remember all of the reasons you started the diet in the first place. The acid alkaline diet isn't an all or nothing diet — it's a continuous process designed to help you on your journey to health.

Working out in a crowd

Here we go again. It's the first week of the new year and the local gym is packed. I can't find a machine that's not occupied, and a crowd of new members is blocking my way to the water cooler. But I'm not stressed. This is a trend I've watched year after year. I know that during the following weeks the new recruits will drop in attendance.

Many people purchase expensive gym memberships (usually attached to a contractual agreement) during or immediately after the winter holidays. Somewhat misguidedly, they hope that the money spent on that membership will be enough motivation to get them to work out routinely. Although working out routinely helps you stabilize weight, no force on earth can get you to the gym if you don't have motivation.

If you want to start working out routinely but don't want to join the ranks of the gym dropouts, you could always start by trying a home workout DVD or taking daily walks. If you can stick with the home routine (and you enjoy it), you may be ready to take the next step and splurge on a commercial gym. It's a matter of personal choice, of course, but I say why waste money if you don't have to? Many of us can get all the physical exercise we need without paying for the expensive equipment and memberships.

Chapter 20

Dealing with Weight Loss Pitfalls

· ·

In This Chapter

▶ Examining weight gain

▶ Looking at good weight loss

▶ Setting goals and shedding pounds

▶ Using a food diary to your advantage

· ·

*I*f the acid alkaline diet is a far cry from your normal fare, your body may not know how to respond initially. You may even *gain* a little weight — just at first, so don't panic. Your weight fluctuates for a number of reasons, some of which are perfectly normal.

A nice side benefit of maintaining the acid alkaline diet is weight loss. Have you ever seen a chunky rabbit? Chances are slim — ha, ha — because it's hard to gain weight when you're munching on healthy, natural foods. But it isn't always easy to lose years of accumulated fluff. This chapter reviews how to set realistic weight loss goals and reach them.

Reviewing Normal Weight Cycles

Whenever you abruptly change your diet, your brain goes into caveman mode. During caveman mode, your metabolism slows to a crawl, and your body hoards every calorie you give it — just in case you're about to starve. It's a prehistoric reflex designed to save your life until your body figures out what's going on.

Take an honest look at your current diet — is it anything similar to the acid alkaline diet? If not, you may be in for a ride while your body adjusts to the invasion of fiber, enzymes, and alkaline-forming foods.

Examining healthy fluctuations

If you've invented colorful words when you step on the scale and see a rise in pounds, you're not alone. Everyone does it (gains weight, not makes up colorful cuss words). Although the human body struggles to keep a fluid balance — what goes in must come out — a fluctuation in daily weight readings is perfectly normal. That weight you gained is not always due to a fat bulge just waiting to appear. Reasons for weight gain after starting a new diet include:

- ✔ Water retention
- ✔ Stool retention from eating more fiber or not drinking enough water
- ✔ Hormonal fluctuations in women (can you say PMS?)

Drink plenty of water while starting the acid alkaline diet to help offset water and stool retention. I also encourage *slowly* increasing the amount of fiber you eat. Going from zero to 60 on the fiber can lead to painful gas, bloating, and constipation.

Tossing your scale out the door

… or window, or whatever portal you can throw it through. Stress hormones are linked to weight gain. I don't know about you, but I get pretty stressed when I step on the scale some days. So I say, toss that scale! Later in this chapter I show you how to take a more realistic (and less stress-producing) measurement of your true weight.

Your body weight is composed of skin, muscles, organs, bones, fluids, and fat. A scale cannot differentiate between the weight of your muscles and the weight of fat. A pound is a pound no matter what substance you're weighing. But I'd personally much rather have pounds of lean muscle mass lining my frame than pounds of fat.

You can start shedding fluff and building lean muscle mass through a combination of cardiovascular exercise (think jogging) and strength training (yes, I mean with actual weights). As you start gaining muscle mass, your weight may be the same on a scale, but your body is healthier because it's muscle, not fat, that your scale is now weighing.

Looking at diets past

Okay, so saying it out loud sounds cheesy, but you have to know where you've been to figure out where you're going. You can gain useful insight by examining the root cause of past failed diets. (I've quit plenty myself, so I'm certainly not labeling anyone as a quitter.)

Can stress really make you fat?

Stress is the archenemy to health. You can blame gray hairs, depression, and even chronic disease on stress. There's one more thing to blame on it — the chunky midsection. This area of your body has more negative slang associated with it than any other part (spare tire, muffin top, inner tube, love handles, scuba tanks — and that's just off the top of my head).

Research shows that people who are chronically stressed tend to have higher levels of the hormone *cortisol* in their bodies. High levels of cortisol can alter blood sugar, metabolism, and even direct where your body stores incoming fat. That's right, high cortisol levels can increase fat storage (including belly fat), which leads to all kinds of health risks including diabetes, stroke, and even heart attack.

A vicious cycle of overeating, fatigue, and more cortisol release ensues if you don't do something to stop the stress. Some ways to cut that worry and regain control of your belly fat include:

✔ Turning off the television. Research shows that folks in developed countries spend way too much time in front of the television; time that could be used for something more mentally or physically stimulating.

✔ Get physical. No matter what exercise you choose, getting physical can boost your mood and combat stress.

✔ Deploy relaxation techniques when you feel that work, responsibility, or any situation is getting out of control. (Chapter 6 offers relaxation tips.)

This isn't a one-size-fits-all strategy — choose something that works for you.

Oftentimes, there are unavoidable reasons to quit a diet. Perhaps it was economically unfeasible, or an illness got you off track. But that's not the norm — most people stop following a diet for one of two reasons (sometimes both):

✔ They didn't feel that it worked.

✔ They got bored with it.

And that's okay. It's human nature to get bored with diets that limit your (insert things you cannot eat here). Fortunately, you don't have to stop eating anything you enjoy, but after you understand how certain foods form acid and what that does to your body, it may be easier to limit or abstain from them altogether.

Oh, and one more groovy thing about eating alkaline-forming foods: You can do it for life. This diet doesn't have an expiration date. Many diets, such as the carb-cutting kind, can have some serious complications if you maintain them for life (your body needs carbohydrates, maybe just not as many as some people eat in a day).

Acidifying Your Body in Fat

Fat is one of the three *macronutrients* (fat, protein, and carbohydrates), which you need to eat to survive. Having said that, many people eat far too much fat every day. It's worse for more than just your waistline — excess fat consumption leads to heart disease, stroke, and it's being linked to certain types of cancer. Fat also has a role in your body's pH balance — it's the acid warehouse. As if you want to save some acids for a rainy day.

How many obese vegetarians do you know? You don't have to go vegetarian, but you can enjoy the health and waistline benefits of decreasing bad fats in your diet by making better food choices.

Fat packs a whopping nine calories per gram (carbs and protein only have four calories per gram). When you eat a fatty food, you're eating twice as many calories as someone enjoying a lean protein or a carbohydrate from a veggie.

Yes, you need fat

Every cell in your body contains fat. It's needed to keep the cellular membrane intact, and it cushions and protects your vital organs. It's also an excellent energy source and allows you to absorb the fat-soluble vitamins A, D, E, and K.

Diets provide three different types of fat:

- ✔ Saturated fat from animal or vegetable sources — the worst type of fat
- ✔ Trans fat, also called partially hydrogenated fat
- ✔ Unsaturated fat, which includes monounsaturated and polyunsaturated fats

The Standard American Diet (SAD), which is typically overloaded with red meats, dairy, and fast food, provides hoards of the two unhealthy fats — saturated and trans fats. The acid alkaline diet, which encourages vegetables and lean proteins, provides healthy fat — unsaturated fat. Unless you're going through a bottle of olive oil a day, it's pretty hard to get too much fat on the acid alkaline diet.

Storing acid for later use

So here's the kicker: High levels of acid in your body make you hold on to fat. A little acid in your bloodstream is usually dumped out through your urine. However, chronically eating acid-forming foods overloads your system, and the excess acids are shipped off to fat cells, where they are stored.

Think of the acid as a car and the fat as a garage. If you keep acquiring cars you need more garages. As long as you keep eating high amounts of acid-forming foods, your body is going to hang on to that fat to keep the acids safely stowed away.

Chronic acidic food ingestion can also lead to one more type of fat storage — a potentially dangerous one called visceral fat. *Visceral fat* is accumulated as your body packs fat around your organs. But it's not simply the result of an acidic diet; other forces increase visceral fat including hormonal fluctuations and stress. It's hard, but not impossible, to lose. You can get started right now by decreasing the need for garages in your body — start decreasing acid-forming foods.

Setting Weight Loss Goals

Yeah, I know you think I took one too many goal-setting seminars in my life by now. The fact remains, the best way to achieve any goal, including weight loss, is by mapping the way to reach it.

Despite the ads that plaster rail-thin models on commercials and magazines, that is not the ideal body. Ideally, you have a healthy amount of lean muscle mass — and no one is meant to look anorexic.

Realizing the unrealistic

At 5'8" I'm never going to be a supermodel for a petite clothing line. The sooner you understand your actual potential and set realistic goals, the sooner you can be at peace with your body shape and start working towards realistic, achievable weight-loss goals.

Rather than arbitrarily saying, "I need to drop about ten pounds," there are several ways to ascertain how much body fat you have:

✔ Use a body mass index (BMI) calculator online. These tools are slightly limited, as they don't account for the amount of lean muscle mass on your frame (athletes may show up in the overweight category), but it's better than a scale.

✔ Get skin caliper measurements. This is a quick, painless way to approximate your body fat percentage. Most personal trainers, and staff members at gyms, universities, and even some physician's offices are trained to use skin calipers and can complete this quick test for you at a minimal fee.

Making it attainable

If your goal is to lose 20 pounds before your best friend's wedding next week, you're out of luck (unless you know a great plastic surgeon and have wads of money). Not only is it nearly impossible to lose 20 pounds in a week, it's unhealthy. Experts agree that you should aim to lose between one and two pounds per week tops. I know that doesn't sound impressive, but if you lose two pounds a week, you could be eight pounds thinner by next month.

Melting Pounds

Literally. When you start to lose weight, your stored fat is liquefied and removed from your body. This can initially cause a rise in your acid output (if you're measuring urine or saliva) as your body breaks down the fat and releases stored acids.

The formula to weight loss isn't a mystery; it's a three-part process:

Diet + Exercise + Overcoming Obstacles = Weight Loss

Weight loss obstacles are frequently overlooked (or sometimes ignored) in the rush to get started on a new diet. A bad knee, veggie aversion, or soda addiction is going to impact your weight loss efforts. To improve your chances (and rate) of success, identify and eliminate your weight loss obstacles before getting started. Bad knee? Go see the doctor and get clearance to exercise or recuperate. Veggie aversion? Slowly immerse your taste buds in new flavors by adding a new vegetable to your diet each week. Soda addiction? Start weaning yourself off the cola and replace it with sparkling mineral water.

Skipping breakfast is a no-no

Skipping breakfast actually slows down your metabolism, which means you burn fewer calories. Your body conserves every calorie just in case you decide not to feed it again during the day. It's like taking a diesel turbo and turning it into a smart car.

Worse yet, skipping meals usually leads to snacking on garbage foods and energy fluctuations throughout the day. When you eat vending machine foods (which are usually high in calories and low in nutrients) your blood sugar spikes — you get that 10 a.m. energy burst and think all is well and good in the world. Come about 11 a.m. your blood sugar drops and suddenly you feel tired, groggy, and irritable. The cycle continues throughout the day or until you feed your body a balanced meal.

It's all right if you're not a breakfast person. Chapter 14 provides plenty of non-breakfast-like foods that can supercharge your day and keep your metabolism running smoothly.

Snacking wisely

Snacks make or break weight loss efforts. A smallish bag of chips (1.5 ounces) and a soft drink can add about 500 calories to your day. Eat it every day and that's 3,500 calories per week, which is equal to about a pound.

Don't forget about the liquid snacks — soda, beer, wine, and other drinks that add empty calories to your diet. They provide zero nutrients and are full of acid-forming sugar. The calories in these beverages quickly add up without providing any feeling of satiety, or fullness.

Snacking is a healthy way to maintain or lose weight — when you snack on the right foods. Whereas the wrong foods just fluff up your waistline, snacking on healthy, alkaline-forming foods benefits your health and keeps you feeling full longer. The next time you need a munchie between mealtimes:

 ✔ Don't wait to eat until you're starving. Eating regular, small snacks throughout the day is a proven way to keep your metabolism revved.

 ✔ Bring healthy snacks with you, at least until vending machines start offering fresh vegetables (wouldn't that be cool).

 ✔ Sip on warm liquids, like vegetable broth, along with water throughout the day to keep hydrated and feel full.

Can you spot the healthy snack?

I am always dumbfounded by the massive display of snacks at the grocery store. If you think about it, the real foods — produce, meat, dairy — usually line the perimeter of the store. The remaining 12 to 20 aisles are stuffed with crackers, chips, sodas, and pre-packaged foods (minus the toilet paper aisle, unless you're a hamster).

So how do you spot the healthiest snack food? If you must venture into the endless rows of snacks, try to remember these tips:

 ✔ Baked, low-fat, and low-calorie don't always mean good for you.

 ✔ Foods with fiber keep you feeling full longer.

 ✔ Check the serving size — many snack foods provide two or more servings in a single pouch.

Don't drink your soup, lift it

Who doesn't want to flaunt their sexy summer arms in a tank top? Although there is no way to lose weight in just one place, like your shoulders, there are ways to tone specific muscles. Toned lean muscles support the skin and help your body burn fat faster (lean muscles require more calories than the rest of your body). You don't need dumbbells or fancy equipment to get started; you need two cans of soup.

A commercial can of soup weighs about a pound. If you're a soup-hater you can substitute two water bottles, which weight about a pound as well. Throughout all of the following exercises be sure to keep your back straight and your neck relaxed:

✔ Warm up your muscles (you get the most benefit from strength workouts if you warm up prior) by taking a brisk five-minute walk or jogging in place.

✔ Sit in a comfortable chair and hold your soup cans at your sides.

✔ Slowly raise your soup cans to your shoulders by flexing at the elbow. You just completed bicep curls! Repeat 10 to 12 times.

✔ Keeping your arms straight, raise your arms until they are level with your shoulders. Repeat 10 to 12 times.

✔ Hold your soup cans level with your shoulders. Raise them straight up over your head, taking heed not to hyperextend your elbows. Repeat 10 to 12 times.

✔ Keeping both arms straight, push your soup cans behind you. Repeat 10 to 12 times.

Controlling your portions

Sad fact: Some people just plain eat too much. Serving sizes have been abandoned like VHS tapes (remember those?). If you're consistently eating calories you don't need, they're consistently turning into unwanted weight.

You need to eat about 3,500 less calories a week to lose one pound. I don't encourage anyone to sit and count every calorie. It's tedious and just encourages you to quit. Just cutting out the additional helpings may get you there!

Even though most alkaline-forming foods are naturally low calorie, you can still go overboard eating too much. This is especially important for your acid-forming foods, like poultry or fish, and for the alkaline-forming foods with healthy fats, such as olive oil, avocadoes, and seeds. A deck of playing cards is about the same size as three ounces of seafood or poultry, and you don't need more than a couple dice worth of fats (seeds, olive oil) per day.

Getting active

Yeah, yeah — I know you've heard it before. Unfortunately, getting active is the answer to stubborn weight problems. Increasing your physical activity has whole-body benefits that can't be faked with a pill or a potion including:

- ✔ Increased and improved circulation. This is the quickest way to get the waste (including acids) filtered out of your body.

- ✔ Decreased blood pressure and work on your heart. The more you exercise the heart (a muscle), the stronger and more efficient it gets.

- ✔ Increased metabolism. Think of it as stoking a fire. The higher you get the flames, the more it consumes. Exercise makes your metabolism go faster, and it burns more calories even when you're doing nothing.

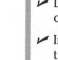

The average person has to hear something between three and seven times before it sinks into their brain. Here goes three: Exercise, exercise, exercise.

Waiting for results

Trying to eat right and exercise and still not seeming to lose weight is a bummer. Since this isn't an infomercial and I'm not wearing spandex, I can safely say that you can lose weight if you stick with a healthy alkaline-forming diet and exercise. However, your health, former activity level, and diet play a role in how quickly you see results.

If you haven't seen any results after a couple months of trying to lose weight, it may be time for a talk with your doctor. He or she can shed light on your personal hurdles and help you refine your weight-loss plan.

Keeping a food diary

It works because it holds you accountable for every morsel. Write down everything (and I mean everything) you put in your mouth. After a week, you may be surprised to find that the "one pretzel" you snack on before lunch actually turns out to be 20 pretzels (it's not your fault that a coworker placed the pretzel jar by the copier).

You're less likely to have that third helping of mashed potatoes if you know you have to write it down in your food journal. For that reason alone, I encourage people who want to lose weight to keep the diary on the refrigerator, in plain sight.

Hurdling Obstacles

I don't know the exact percentage, but for a small population, the weight-loss tactics mentioned in the preceding sections don't work. Hormone imbalances, chronic disease, and even familial genes can inhibit your best efforts.

Frequently, people get off track with weight loss due to a physical situation that makes it challenging, such as:

- **Chronic back, neck, or knee problems:** Ask your doctor if physical therapy would be of benefit. A physical therapist can help you develop an exercise program that is safe.

- **Chronic pain:** It's extremely difficult to exercise with pain. Ask your doctor if swimming is allowed. Many people report decreased pain in the buoyancy of the water.

- **Fatigue:** An exercise buddy may help encourage you and keep both of you motivated.

Considering special situations

The guidelines I provide for weight loss are intended for the average healthy adult — period. Certain people should always consult with a doctor before attempting to cut calories or lose weight including:

- Children and the elderly
- Pregnant or nursing women
- Person with a chronic illness of any kind
- Person recovering from an illness or surgery
- Athletes

I would need to devote an entire book to the intricacies of diet, nutrition, and weight loss within each of these very special populations.

Chapter 21

Finding Support

I'm not talking about the fit of your panty hose; I'm talking about feeling unsupported while making dietary and lifestyle changes. Beginning a new diet is challenging under any circumstances. But when the diet involves a little chemistry and know-how about your body, it can be daunting.

But I have very reassuring news: Quite honestly, you cannot screw up on this diet. You may always have room for improvement in the form of an even better pH balance, but even switching a soda for a glass of lemon water is a great start.

This chapter gives you the tools to rebuke criticism of your dietary choices (for reasons unknown to me, the acid alkaline diet still isn't a common household term). I've compiled Internet do's and don'ts, as well as ways to find professional support while showing you how to avoid Internet scams.

Do you have picky eaters in your family? As long as you aren't making them pH test their urine (that's awkward), there's no reason why your children can't enjoy healthy, alkaline-forming foods. So if you have children, a partner, or even a table-scrap-eating dog, this chapter shows you how to get the entire family on board with your alkaline eating plan.

Dealing with Criticism

Face it: You're going to get criticized at some point. Could be someone doesn't like your political views, the shirt you're wearing, or someone who doesn't understand your dietary choices. Unless the criticizer is your Higher Power or your physician, my advice is to invest in a good pair of earplugs and use them. Okay, so you would look goofy wearing earplugs all the time, but the point is — don't listen.

Demystifying the diet

The biggest obstacle I've overcome is the fact that many people don't understand what a pH balanced diet is. This lack of knowledge sometimes leads to avoidance, suspicion, and criticism.

Without getting into the nitty gritty by the water cooler at your office, there's a pretty straightforward way to explain a pH balanced diet: Eating a diet composed mostly of healthy, fresh foods helps your body maintain health. End of subject.

Exposing the myths

Many myths surround the acid alkaline diet, most of which are false (and some are just plain ridiculous). Following are the top five myths that you may come across:

- ✔ "It's impossible to control your pH balance."

  Um, no, it's not. Although you cannot control the pH balance of your blood, you can control the amount of acid floating throughout your body and impact your pH through diet, exercise, and even mood control.

- ✔ "You can only eat rabbit foods on that diet."

  Again false. There is nothing wrong with eating low-fat animal proteins, as long as you keep them in moderation and balance them with natural, alkaline-forming foods.

- ✔ "The acid alkaline diet is too strict. You can't eat (insert favorite food here) anymore."

  Actually, a pH balanced diet is extremely flexible. You don't have to count every calorie, weigh portions, or suffer prepackaged meals. You can eat a variety of healthy foods while still enjoying the occasional acid-forming food.

- ✔ "Those diets are expensive."

  Not any more so than any other healthy, balanced diet. Sure, it would be less expensive to live on tuna fish and bananas, but what kind of nutrition would that provide?

- ✔ "That's a fad diet and it doesn't work."

  Define work, please. The acid alkaline diet is not a trendy fad, it's a way to promote health and wellness by helping your body function at its peak.

Beware: Outrageous fad diets back in favor

The term *fad diet* is urban slang, loosely defined as a diet that is largely popular, but doesn't survive the test of time. I've looked far and wide for the craziest dieting trends over the past decade. And the top five winners are . . .

✔ **The Grapefruit Diet:** As long as you eat a grapefruit with every meal, you can fry up other foods and eat all the cholesterol you like. Hmm, sounds too good to be true, anyone?

✔ **The Juice Fast Diet:** You abstain from foods and drink a special juice for two days or so. Purportedly you'll lose about ten pounds. What do you think is going to happen when you start eating real food again? (That's assuming that you don't pass out from low blood sugar in the meantime.)

✔ **The Baby Food Diet:** On this diet, you eat nothing but baby food. Apologize to your colon now, because as an adult, baby foods probably won't meet your required grams of fiber or calories for any given day.

✔ **The Cabbage Soup Diet:** Ever read a Harlequin romance? This fad's been around for a century at least. The romantics called it a "reducing" diet. You eat nothing but cabbage soup and lose weight. Yum. (Not.)

✔ **The Tapeworm Diet:** Just plain disgusting, it is what it sounds like. You intentionally infect yourself with tapeworms (have you ever seen one?) to induce a state of malnutrition and lose weight.

Locating Support Near You

It's a proven fact that many diets work because they provide a network of social support. The key to a good support system revolves around finding like-minded people. If I look at five people who purchase this book, I bet at least two have similar goals in mind. If you want to lose weight, find a weight-loss support group. If you want to be mindful of your health, find a health support group. And if you're an introvert, don't worry, you can locate plenty of web-based support groups.

Finding a nutritionist

There's no doubt that talking to a health care professional can provide support, answers, and help along your pH balanced journey. Consider the following health care professionals who specialize in nutrition:

✔ **Registered Dietitian (RD):** This is the golden standard for a nutritionist. He or she has completed at least a baccalaureate and is a licensed professional.

✔ **Certified Dietetic Nutritionist** and **Certified Nutrition Specialist:** A person with one of these credentials completes an associates or bachelor's degree within the field and has passed a certification examination.

✓ **Dietetic Nutritionist, Nutritionist,** or **Dietary Manager:** A nutritionist completes an associates or bachelor's degree within the field, but does not take a certification examination. Many states restrict the practice of nutritionists who do not hold a certification or license.

Finding the right person can get a little tricky, especially considering the alphabet soup of titles for nutritionists. For more information on researching health professionals, visit the website for the Academy of Nutrition and Dietetics at www.eatright.org.

Or you can look up your local health department, health regulation agency, or simply ask your doctor. He or she can show you how to tailor nutritional needs and provide a referral for (or at least offer a way to contact) a licensed nutrition specialist.

Avoiding online scams

Unfortunately, some online pH balancing sites are overloaded with biased information and claims intended to sell a product. If you choose to do online research or purchase an "alkalinizing" supplement, be sure to research the company's reputation and check if there's any scientific evidence backing up the products and claims.

It's best to avoid any website that:

✓ Promises unrealistic or amazing results, especially fast.

✓ Encourages you to eliminate entire food groups.

✓ Claims that you do not need to exercise or make any behavior modifications on your part because their product does all the work.

✓ Doesn't back up products with links to quality research. Many sites provide one or two small studies to back up a product, which are conducted by the manufacturer of said product.

Spotting a quality resource

I'm not stating that everyone trying to sell a product online is a phony. I am saying that you have to use the common-sense check before buying into the fabulous claims of many pH diet supporters. Some acid alkaline websites, while intended to help you, may actually provide misleading information.

When you seek quality, science-based information, it's best to turn to the non-profit, governmental, and university sponsored websites. These sites usually end in:

> ✔ .org
> ✔ .edu
> ✔ .gov

Expensive supplements and other products (water ionizers, pH drops, food dehydrators) are nice, but they are not essential to enjoy an acid alkaline diet. I mention this only because so many pH resources (both online and written texts) are going to refer you back to these extraneous items.

Involving the Family

It's no fun making two or three different meals every night, just as it's no fun to make the kids French fries and avoid their salty allure because you're trying to eat better. The solution is simple: Don't. Don't cook different foods for everyone at your dinner table.

The entire family can eat an acid alkaline diet. It doesn't restrict food groups or severely limit calories (drastically cutting calories can be dangerous for some people). Plus, a diet centering on vegetables and healthy proteins can benefit everyone in your household.

Dieting and kids

If getting kids to eat right were easy, there wouldn't be hundreds of books showing you how to hide, evade, and basically trick youngsters into eating healthy foods. Younger children may not be able to grasp the concept of pH balance, but they can start appreciating the fact that food is fuel — and that there's good fuel and bad fuel. If you have older children, consider explaining the acid alkaline diet to them as well as your rationale for starting it. Middle and high schoolers may get a kick out of the chemistry involved and become your biggest supporters.

Do not put your children on a calorie-restrictive diet unless your physician has instructed you to do so. Do show them how to balance their plates with healthy, natural foods and lean, muscle-building proteins.

Making it fun

Yes, that *is* spinach on your plate. No, it won't crawl off on its own. Children of all ages love to touch, taste, and smell everything. If you put a green blob of food in front of them, chances are they'll automatically dismiss it as disgusting. Half the battle is getting your kids to try new foods.

A very real problem: Obesity and children

Obesity is defined as having excess percentage of body fat for your height, which can lead to a number of chronic diseases. The past few decades have introduced an alarming statistic — the number of obese children is on the rise. Some people think belly rolls or chubby cheeks are cute, but these children may be at serious risk for adult diseases. Obese children are susceptible to type 2 diabetes, high blood pressure, and even hormonal imbalances that can lead to an early onset of puberty. Worse yet, these children can suffer problems with self-esteem that will follow them into their adult lives.

Experts agree that although some obese children may have predisposing factors, such as genetic diseases, the majority of children are not exercising enough and are eating a poor diet.

Some kids grow into their weight or simply have large frames for their age; these children are not obese. Only your doctor can tell if your child is at risk, so make an appointment if you're concerned about your child's health.

You can win the battle for your kids' palates by embracing their senses:

- ✔ **Sight:** Talk about the different colors, shapes, and sizes of natural foods. Cut foods into fun shapes, and arrange at least three different colored foods on each plate.

- ✔ **Hearing:** Listen to the peas snap as you prepare them. Turn off the television, and play quiet music at meal time.

- ✔ **Smell:** Zest a lemon together, and encourage identifying healthy foods by smell. Plant an herb garden, and encourage children to smell the different bouquets.

- ✔ **Touch:** Show them how to wash and peel fruits and vegetables. Teach them how to pick fresh produce based on texture and feel.

- ✔ **Taste:** Pair healthy foods with creamy dips. Encourage a little bite of healthy foods at every meal.

Use these tips to win over hearts in the kitchen.

Eating in a rush

Everyone has done that thing where you stand in the kitchen and inhale a sandwich, and everyone knows that doing that isn't good for your digestion. I know all about responsibilities and trying to rush kids off to sports, but the quick grab-and-go meals are not conducive to good digestion — for you or your kids.

You can cause stress in your body every time you gobble down food standing at the counter and don't take the time to sit and relax. Shuffle things around in your schedule and make the time to sit down and eat.

Whenever you become stressed — even just a little — your saliva dries up and the blood supply to your digestive organs (stomach, intestines, kidneys, and so on) shuts off. This is part of your nervous system known as the *fight-or-flight response,* or how your body prepares itself to defend against danger (real or imagined). Honestly, who needs spit or stomach juice when they're about to be attacked?

The fight-or-flight response does things like increase your heart rate to shuttle more blood to your muscles for action and dilates your pupils to give you more light to see better and fight.

Although it's meant to protect you from danger, the fight-or-flight response has the unfortunate side effect of slowing your food digestion. This is especially bad when you eat acid-forming foods, because they stay in your stomach and intestines longer.

Help your body digest its food by:

- ✔ Sitting down and relaxing during a meal.
- ✔ Taking small bites and chewing thoroughly.
- ✔ Sipping a beverage throughout the meal.
- ✔ Paying attention to flavors and textures (forces you to slow down).

Feeding picky eaters

"I'm not eating that." If every meal with your children feels like a war of wills, it might be time to regain control of their diet. There's a good chance Tommy will grow out of eating nothing but macaroni and hot dogs, but as his parent, you can help him out of that rut.

Chances are, you're going to have to put a new food on your child's plate more than once before she accepts it. My children turned up their noses at tofu the first three times I made it. The fourth time they sampled it and the fifth time they asked for it (not by name, they called it "that white stuff"). You're going to need a stronger will than that of your children, as well as a little patience.

Finding the Ingredients

Regardless of where you live, sometimes finding the right ingredients is a challenge. Larger cities may have an abundance of health food stores, but few produce stands. Likewise, you may have a fresh produce stand down the street in a small town, but no access some gourmet alkaline foods, such as barley or spelt pasta.

Markets and what you can probably find there include

- **Traditional grocery store:** You can find the acid alkaline diet staples, such as fresh vegetables, in the produce section. Larger chains usually boast a health food section in the produce or dairy aisle, where tofu, soy, or almond milk (and yogurt) and sprouted grains are found. Silken tofu does not need to be refrigerated until it's opened, so you may find that in a center aisle or health food aisle.

- **Farmers market or produce stand:** Visiting the local stand is an excellent way to find new fruits and vegetables. Since these products are locally grown, you can learn what produce is in season and try exploring new flavors for a reasonable price. Some markets include vendors who supply fruits and fruit products, farm-fresh eggs, fish, salmon, and even organic honey.

- **Health food store:** This is where I usually discover the gourmet alkaline-forming foods, such as spelt pasta, sprouted grain products, and yeast-free vegetable broths. Many health-food chain stores have an amazing produce section where you can find fruits and vegetables from around the world and expand your palate's culture. You may also find the more exotic alkaline-friendly ingredients here, such as almond or spelt flour and seaweed.

Shopping online for hard-to-find foods

You may not have access to health food stores or anything more than a traditional grocery store without (gasp) a health food section. Never to fear — go there to buy your lean proteins (skinless chicken, fish), vegetables, fruits and acid-forming foods. The rest of your shopping can be completed online.

You have the option of going straight to the product's website and ordering it direct, or you can find retailers online and shop for multiple items. Sprouted grain products, gourmet sea salt, and spelt pastas are available on the web and are some of the harder alkaline diet items to find in traditional stores. To get you started:

- For **gourmet sea salt,** you can visit www.saltworks.us/gourmet-sea-salt.asp and pick the flavor or consistency that appeals to you.

✔ For **spelt pasta varieties,** go to www.plummarket.com and plug spelt pasta into the search window.

✔ For **sprouted grain breads,** type sprouted grain bread into your favorite search engine and choose from the numerous retailers.

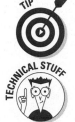

If you know you like a product and want to order it online, I suggest ordering in bulk quantity to save on shipping costs (and to keep your cupboard full of a healthy favorite).

You can order most perishable products on the web, such as cream cheese or meat replacements. They arrive packed in dry ice and can slip right into your refrigerator or freezer!

Growing your own

I really encourage this option, especially if you have a big yard. It's so easy to grow produce, and many of the plants provide an inexhaustible source of fresh herbs and vegetables. (Plus, it'll cut down on the amount of grass you have to mow each week.)

If you have no experience growing edible plants, here are some pointers to get started:

✔ Start with one or two vegetables or herbs that you use frequently in the kitchen. (I started with basil, because it's a versatile herb that can be used on almost everything, and jalapenos.)

✔ Grow things in pots in sunny windows if you live in an apartment or condo. Remember to get pots with holes in the bottom, and place trays underneath them (it's hard to over-water them that way).

✔ Don't use heavy-duty or flowering plant pesticides on plants that produce edible food. Read the labels and ask someone at your local nursery. Also, if pests become problematic, collect one in a jar and bring it to the nursery experts. They can provide a safe organic option for pest removal.

✔ Watch your plants. Problems are usually easy to correct if you catch them early. For instance, leaves start to turn yellowish when you over-water.

✔ Place cinnamon sticks, bay leaves, or coffee grounds around your garden if you don't like the ants coming near. They hate the smell.

✔ Freeze your new produce if you are plucking more than you can use.

Most importantly, have fun with it. Before I got good at gardening, I once killed a cactus (true story).

Part VI
The Part of Tens

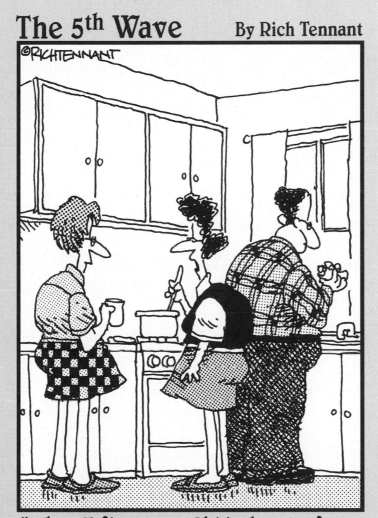

The 5th Wave   By Rich Tennant

"When I first met Philip, he ate from the Food Guide Stonehenge. It was a mysterious diet and no one's sure what its purpose was."

In this part...

The following chapters are stuffed with quick tips for the acid alkaline diet. If you're a bottom-line kind of person, you're going to love this part. I present the top ten foods to avoid at all cost and I even tell you why. Or, if you're not ready for that, you can skip to the chapter on lifestyle changes and the best ways to embrace pH living or read how to exchange some common acid-forming foods for more alkaline-friendly choices. You're welcome.

Chapter 22

Ten Worst Foods for pH Balance

In This Chapter
▶ Discovering which foods to banish altogether
▶ Uncovering the ugly truth about certain ingredients
▶ Realizing how many foods incorporate acid-forming substances

*I*f you aren't ready to put forth the effort to begin an acid alkaline lifestyle right now but you want to start eating better for your pH, this chapter lists the ten worst acid-forming foods, ingredients, and beverages in a few succinct pages.

You can make this your do-not-buy grocery list or your avoid-at-all-costs restaurant menu guide. However you choose to use this list, these ten items are some of the worst pH wreckers I've found. (Don't worry, if you skip ahead to Chapter 24 I'll show you how to exchange some of these foods with more wholesome, alkaline-forming foods.)

It's not the pH of the food as it goes in that you have to worry about. Your pH is affected during digestion, when foods leave an acidic ash in your digestive tract.

Beef

Hamburger, steak, and chuck roast are all acid-forming meats. Animal flesh of any kind is acid-forming in your body, but some animal proteins, like poultry, are less offensive to your pH than red and processed meat. Beef is by far the biggest offender.

You can't skate around the fact that animal flesh contains acid — when you eat the animal flesh it forms acidic ash in your digestive tract (not to mention that red and processed meat is also proven to increase your risk of colorectal cancer). It doesn't matter what part of the cow you eat, all cuts will bottom out your pH.

Artificial Sweeteners

Actually I think artificial sweeteners should be tied with beef for first place in the worst acid-forming category. Artificial sweeteners are chemical food additives — they may look (somewhat) like sugar and taste (somewhat) like sugar, but they aren't sugar. These food additives are found in many diet and low-calorie products and are extremely acid-forming during digestion. Check the ingredients for sucralose, saccharin, aspartame, and acesulfame potassium — they're all artificial sweeteners.

Fried Foods

To uncover the reason why fried foods are so bad for your pH, you have to examine how food is fried. You take the food, dip it in egg, milk, or both (both are acid-forming), dip it in a batter preparation (usually a mixture of refined flour and seasonings — again, acid-forming) and fry it in a bath of trans or saturated fats — your third acid strike. After the food gets nice and crispy — think French fries — you'll probably want to dip it in something to further boost the flavor (think acid-forming ketchup). It's a virtual acid pile-up on your road to a healthier pH.

Trans fat and saturated fat are by far two of the worst things you can feed your body. They increase your bad cholesterol, your weight, and raise your risk for heart attack and stroke. These fats are hidden in commercialized products like donuts, some margarines, and even cooking oils.

Sugary Delights

Sugar is a highly acid-forming ingredient found in so many different substances we eat. I could make this entire list out of foods containing sugar, but I thought that might get a bit tedious.

Everyone knows that eating too much sugar can increase your waistline, but did you know that it can also increase your chance of developing diabetes? That's not a myth, it's a fact. When you chronically ingest too much sugar (think daily sodas), your pancreas has to work overtime to regulate the sugar in your blood stream. This sometimes leads to a condition called *insulin resistance*, which is a precursor to type 2 diabetes. When your body becomes insulin resistant, it gets used to the overload of sugar and stops working as hard to combat it. This causes your sugar-regulating hormone, insulin, to become less effective and your blood sugar levels remain elevated.

High blood sugar can lead to all kinds of chronic disease, not just an acidic pH. Think about how much sugar you consume daily in the form of colas, fruit juices, sweets, and treats — then consider what it's doing to your pH.

Ice Cream

I scream, you scream, we all scream for . . . high cholesterol? I know, I know, it's absolutely delicious and refreshing on a hot, summer day, but ice cream takes the prize as the worst dairy product for your pH. It includes a mixture of acid-forming dairy products, such as milk fat, and pairs it with sugar and more saturated fat. Some old-fashioned recipes even call for egg yolks to give it that creamy texture when it melts, but now most commercial products use an equally acid-forming ingredient of trans or saturated fats.

If you want to cool off and save your body from acid overload, suck on some fruit-juice flavored ice and leave the frozen fats for someone else.

Commercially Baked Goods

Donuts, bread, cake, cookies — pretty much anything you lay eyes on behind that bakery glass falls into this category. If you didn't make it yourself, you don't know what's in it. Acid-forming yeast and refined flour are two of the biggest culprits that put commercially baked goods on the do-not-eat list.

Don't be fooled by the commercial goods made for diabetics. Most simply exchange real sugar for fake sugar, which is still acid-forming.

Beer and Other Alcohol

What if I offered you an iced mug full of sugar and fermented yeast? Beer is composed of yeast, hops, malted grains, sugar, and sometimes salt. It's not only the ethanol that acidifies your pH, it's all of the ingredients! And it's not just beer (sorry) but all forms of ethanol (alcohol) that drop your pH. Wine, grain alcohol, beer — you name it.

If you drink alcohol, remember to stick to the suggested daily serving size, which is one to two drinks for men and one drink for women. Oh, and a drink is about 12 ounces of beer, 5 ounces of wine and an ounce and a half of spirits. Oops, that fishbowl-sized margarita you had with dinner probably provided about four times the recommended alcohol intake, which means about four times the acid, as well.

Lobster

Sorry, Maine, but this delightful crustacean is one of the most acid-forming shellfish around. Lobster — and sardines, mussels, and anchovies — are full of protein and a substance called purine. *Purine* is a chemical compound that's turned into uric acid following digestion. A little uric acid in your system is okay, which is a good thing because many foods contain purine. However, a lot of uric acid in your body not only tips your personal pH scale, it can build up in your joints and cause a painful condition called *gout*.

Condiments

Like I say in Chapter 9, the majority of your acid-forming foods are hiding on the shelf of your refrigerator. Whether it comes in a single-use packet, glass jar, or a convenient squeeze bottle, condiments wreck your pH. Worse yet, they're usually hiding in almost every fast food on the menu.

Give your taste buds a little time to adjust. Once you stop drenching your foods in ketchup or suffocating salads in fatty dressings, your mouth may actually start to appreciate the myriad natural flavors of the foods.

Starchy Veggies

If you were having a conversation with your stomach, starch is just another name for sugar. Starchy veggies are sugary veggies (probably why they taste so great). Avoid or limit these pH wreckers that include white potatoes, corn, peas, acorn squash, and parsnips.

Chapter 23

Top Ten Ways to Embrace pH Balance

In This Chapter

▶ Examining your diet

▶ Reducing your acids and your stress

▶ Jumping onto the exercise train

*W*hat the acid alkaline diet is: A way to manage your nutrition, health and well-being through food. What it isn't: A fad to help you drop ten pounds before that wedding next month. Your pH balance is not just about what you eat and drink — if only it were that easy. A pH-balanced body requires a pH-balanced life. Sure, you'll benefit from eating an acid alkaline diet, but you'll really benefit from cutting out all the other garbage that causes acid build-up as well.

I condensed every bit of pH-enhancing wisdom I have into this one, tiny chapter. Of course there's a couple food tips, but the rest of the pearls are things you may not even be thinking about when you ponder balancing your pH.

Controlling the Carnivore

And by carnivore I don't just mean meat eater — I mean eater of anything that comes from an animal. Limiting your animal protein intake is probably the easiest way to help boost your pH back into alkaline territory, where your body is the happiest (and functions most efficiently).

As you switch to an acid-reducing, alkaline-enhancing diet, you don't have to completely stop eating and drinking all of the things you love, you just have to limit them and add more alkaline-forming foods to your diet. (Chapter 11 talks about foods good and bad for your pH levels.) That applies especially to red and processed meats and dairy (think moo cow) products, which you should severely limit or avoid altogether. They wreck your pH and leave acidic ash in your digestive tract.

Boosting the Veggies

Think back to your last plate of food. How much of it was covered in fresh fruit or vegetables? (French fries don't count.) If you up your veggie intake at each meal, you're automatically adding alkaline-forming foods to your diet.

A good rule: For every one part meat or protein sitting on your plate, combat it's acidity with at least three parts fruit or vegetable. This way, you're eating at least 75 percent alkalinizing foods and only 25 percent acid-forming ones without even pulling out a scale or measuring cup!

Eating Natural

Bags of chips don't grow on trees, and chocolate candies don't grow in your garden (unless you're Willy Wonka). Eat as many foods as you can in their natural form. Follow this rule around snack time to help limit your choices to healthier options. If it doesn't grow in the earth, it's probably not your best pH bet. (And if you locate a cheese doodle tree, please give me a call!)

It's not just the processed food that's bad for your pH, it's also the preservatives and artificial additives that sneak in there and potentially harm your body's cellular pH balance.

Drinking Your Water

Okay it's gross, but imagine your home plumbing system without any water. How exactly would that work? Fact is, it wouldn't, and neither does your body. You can eat all the healthy, alkaline-forming foods you want, but if you don't give the acid fluid to ride out on, it's going to take up residence in your cells.

Try to drink at least half your pounds of body weight in ounces of fresh water daily. (A 100 pound person needs at least 50 ounces of water, which translates to just over six 8-ounce glasses.) The water transports garbage out of your body and keeps your tissues plump and happy (in a good way — think grapes, not raisins).

Taking a Deep Breath

Like, right now. Breathe in through your nose for a count of five seconds and out through your mouth for five seconds . . . doesn't that feel better? You just forced carbonic acids out of your body through a little lung work.

I find it funny that almost everyone I know takes breathing for granted. It's one of the only life-sustaining functions that you can control, but you don't have to. It's also one of the quickest ways to force acids out and achieve a level of calm.

A chronically stressed person is probably a chronically acidic one. Don't let negative emotions rule you; discover how to control and manage your emotions — your pH thanks you.

Going for a Walk

And consider making it a part of your daily routine. Seriously, if you haven't used those sticks holding up your body today, step outside and at least get to the mailbox and back.

Daily exercise is great for your pH balance (and your heart, muscles, bones and pretty much every gooey substance inside you). Any cardiovascular activity that gets blood pumping throughout your body helps flush trapped acids from pockets of fat. It takes time, but someone who exercises routinely is going to see a benefit in the form of his or her alkaline pH. (I talk about the exercise-pH connection in Chapter 6.)

Cutting Out the Stimulants

Yep, I love my cup of java, too, but it may be holding back your pH balance. Stimulants and drugs like nicotine and caffeine acidify your cells. The majority of the beverages containing caffeine have absolutely no nutritional value and are a sugary transport for the stimulant.

If you smoke, chew tobacco, or use any kind of nicotine product, you may want to look into cessation classes before you start your acid alkaline diet. The nicotine can combat your alkalinizing efforts. It's like adding vitamins and fiber to a bucket of ice cream — in the end, it's still a bucket of ice cream. The nicotine can negate your alkalinizing choices, so try to quit.

Reading Labels

I know it sounds ridiculously obvious, but this is probably the most important thing you can do at the grocery store. You only know what's in that freezer meal or canned good by reading the food label. The good news — natural foods don't need labels (when's the last time you saw a list of ingredients on an apple?), but processed and preserved foods do.

If you can't pronounce 90 percent of the ingredients, there's a really good chance that the food choice is acid-forming.

Being a Savvy Shopper

Bottom line: Don't shop when you're hungry, always carry a list, and try to avoid the aisles. On the acid alkaline diet, the majority of your ingredients are found in the produce section, which is usually somewhere on the perimeter of the store away from the aisles packed with the packaged and processed foods.

Planning your weekly meals ahead of time (and even cooking them) helps lower the chances that you'll cheat and sneak a pH-lowering pizza or burger during a busy week. (I offer shopping tips in Chapter 13.)

Keeping an Open Mind

If you enter this diet believing you will fail, guess what? You will fail. The acid alkaline diet is not a hip trend — it's a way of life and healthy nutrition that can help you regain balance within your body.

Not to sound too Zen, but everything in life has a proper balance and order. To good there is evil, to night there is day, and to acid there is alkaline. Don't quit if you cheat, and don't get discouraged if you see nothing but acidic pH results in the beginning — maintaining your health is a marathon, not a sprint.

Chapter 24

Top Ten Acid Alkaline Swaps (Eat This, Not That)

. . . .

In This Chapter

▶ Swapping out acidic choices

▶ Getting creative in the kitchen

. . . .

Adhering to your acid alkaline diet can be challenging when you don't have the right ingredients on hand. A little cheat with sugar here, a little cheat with flour there — before you know it, all of those acid-forming cheats start to add up. In this chapter, I provide some alkalinizing swaps you can use instead of the ten highly acid-forming ingredients usually found in classic recipes.

Didn't get to the store this week? No problem. Eat this, not that, and you'll stay on the road to an alkaline pH.

Tofu for Beef

Now don't go wrinkling up your nose, tofu is the master magician of proteins. It can be chicken, beef, or even vegetable flavored, depending on how you sauté it. Fact is firm tofu has virtually no flavor. It takes on the flavors of the dish. If you press it nice and dry before cooking (or freeze it for a day) it takes on a meaty, chewy quality that can replace animal flesh in almost any dish.

Don't discount tofu for eggs, either. Crumbled tofu can be used in placed of scrambled eggs in casseroles. Sprinkle it with some turmeric if you crave the egg-like appearance — it colors your tofu and tricks your peepers.

Honey for Sugar

When you need to make a dish or beverage sweet, think about using clover honey (the real deal, not the processed dime-a-dozen bottles). Some experts argue that honey is mildly acid-forming, but it's still far less so than cane sugar, high-fructose corn syrup, or the chemicals in artificial sweeteners.

Raw honey is a wee bit sweeter than sugar; you'll have to play with your recipes until you get the conversion right. Since it's a liquid, you also might want to decrease your other liquid ingredients a smidgen so you don't end up with runny baked goods (who wants a runny cookie?)

Olive Oil for Shortening

Cold-pressed olive oil can be substituted for acid-forming cooking fats (shortening, for example) in most recipes without impacting the taste of the dish. Think about what you use lard or hydrogenated oils for . . . to fry things, right? Since you don't fry anything on the acid alkaline diet, you can just drop those artery-clogging lards altogether.

I've watched a frightening new trend develop — the use of palm kernel oil for cooking. It's scary that this tropical oil is being promoted as a healthy alternative to vegetable oil when it's loaded with saturated fat (the bad kind).

Vegetable Stock for Bouillon

The next time a recipe calls for beef or chicken stock or bouillon, consider using yeast-free vegetable stock instead. Meat-based broths are just as acid-forming as the meats they're made from. The conversion doesn't take any culinary expertise; exchange the vegetable stock for the meat stock at a 1:1 ratio.

Chapter 14 contains some tips on making and storing your own vegetable base, so you are no longer held hostage to looking for a can of yeast-free broth.

Almonds for Flour

No, I haven't lost my marbles. You can use ground natural almonds (almond flour or meal) in place of acid-forming refined flour in many recipes.

Don't use salted or processed almonds. If you want to make your own almond flour, purchase natural blanched or unblanched almonds. (Blanched just means that their skin has been removed.)

All you need to make your own almond flour is a coffee bean grinder and a sifter. But don't forget to store your almond meal in the refrigerator; it can go bad if you leave it out (no preservatives means a short shelf life).

Mashed Veggies for Thickness

Prior to giving a hoot about my pH, I would use whatever I had on hand to thicken sauces, soups, and stews. However, traditional thickening agents include ingredients like refined flour, cornstarch, and gelatin. Unfortunately, all three of these products are extremely acidifying and make your pH plummet.

Try adding some extra veggies to your recipe and gently mashing them to add thickness. Cauliflower works great in many dishes and it doesn't impart much flavor once cooked. For sauces and soups, you can also crank down the heat and let it simmer longer. The fluids will eventually evaporate, leaving a thicker base to work with.

Sprouted Grains for Wheat

Don't knock it till you try it! Any refined grain product (bread, tortillas) is acid-forming during digestion. Sprouted grain products are alkalinizing during digestion — the sprouts add antioxidants to your diet and help your body retain alkaline-forming minerals.

Sprouted grain products are available at health food stores (you can some-times find them in the health food section of well-established grocery chains). I've found sprouted grain bread, tortillas, rolls, and even muffins online. They're a bit chewier than regular refined grain products, but I find they're also far more satisfying.

Sea Salt for Table Salt

Isn't salt, salt? Nope, it's not. Sea salt is formed from an evaporative process, not a chemical one. The minerals and flavor of the sea salt come from the seawater where it was harvested. It comes in many different sizes, colors, and even tastes. On the other hand, those tiny, uniform granules of refined table salt are nothing more than chemically altered molecules from salt mines.

Sea salt is alkaline-forming because of its rich mineral content. Ditch the shaker, and pick up the grinder!

Green Tea for Coffee

Okay, so it's not an ingredient, per say, but I had to include it. It kills me to say this, but coffee (that includes espresso, mocha, you name it) is acidifying. Got a hankering for a hot beverage? Try swapping out your java for a cleansing cup of green tea. Green tea is packed with antioxidants — the healthy little compounds that clean toxins out of your system. You can choose an herbal tea if you prefer (and you can even make your own by steeping the herb of your choice).

I have yet to try it, but some people advocate that cold-pressed coffee is less acid-forming than a hot brew. The premise lies with the fact that heating the ground beans releases more acid.

Clarified Butter for Fats

When a recipe calls for butter or margarine, you can use the clarified butter recipe I provide in Chapter 13. Clarified butter, also known as *ghee,* provides the lubricants without the acidifying milk fats associated with butter (or the chemicals associated with margarine).

Ghee works well in baked goods, oven dishes, and even the occasional sautéed dish (although I prefer to use cold-pressed olive oil for sautés). Prime ghee should be a translucent golden yellow without any solids.

Part VII
Appendixes

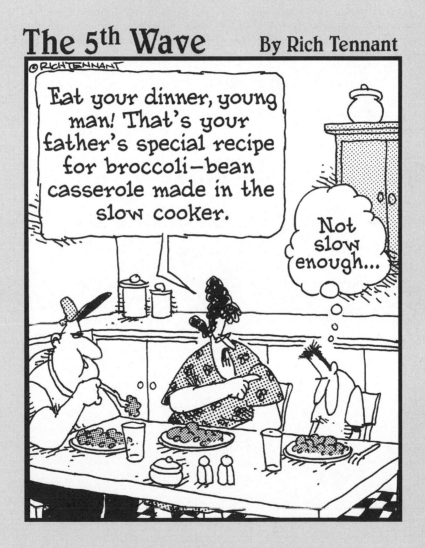

In this part...

This brief part contains two handy reference tools. In the first one, I provide a list of common acid-forming foods and ingredients along with some alkaline-friendly exchanges. There's nothing worse than being stuck halfway through cooking a dish because you're unsure what ingredients to use.

The second appendix provides a convenient list of metric conversions that allow all of us to speak a common measurement language. Based on personal experience, a recipe can take a real bad turn on your taste buds if you don't use the right measurements!

Substitute Foods for Better pH Choices

The acid alkaline diet boils down to choices. Your pH hinges on every choice you make. Do you put two spoonfuls of sugar in the tea or use a dollop of fresh honey? It's your choice — and your pH. Use this appendix as a kitchen cheat sheet. You won't always have alkaline-forming ingredients on hand, but if you want to use a more alkaline-forming (or less acid-forming) substitute, you can probably find it here, in these pages.

I don't want to read paragraphs of information scanning for a quick answer, and I'm sure you don't either. That's why I arranged this appendix in easy-to-use tables. I've grouped foods and beverages into their own tables, similar to how they are arranged in cookbooks (beverages, meats, vegetables, and so on). My editor (not my OCD) made me put them in alphabetical order.

Common Baking Ingredients

If you're up for experimenting, you can replace some of the more common ingredients in your baked goods for alkaline-forming ones. Gelatin, for instance, is made from animal byproducts and is an extremely acid-forming thickener. Table A-1 shows some common exchanges to use while making your favorite delectable.

Table A-1	Ingredient Substitutions for Baked Goods
Instead of This...	*...Use This*
Butter	Clarified butter
Eggs	Egg whites, silken tofu, egg replacements
Fillings (pie, puddings, fruit)	Real fruit, silken tofu
Wheat flour	Almond flour, spelt flour
Gelatin	Agar-agar, arrowroot
Sugar	Honey, stevia
Syrup	Honey, stevia, molasses
Yeast	Baking soda

Beans

Regardless of the type, beans are a better source of lean protein for your pH than animal protein. However, certain beans are more alkaline-forming, such as lentils, and can be substituted for the less alkaline-forming legumes, such as pinto beans, in almost any recipe. Table A-2 shows ideas for exchanging legumes within your favorite dishes.

Table A-2	Beans
Instead of This...	*Use This...*
Chili beans (canned)	Kidney beans
Navy beans	Black-eyed peas
Pinto, split pea, or white beans	Lentils (red or brown)
Refried beans (canned)	Black-eyed peas, black beans

Beverages

Before you pop the top on that cold refreshment, know that beverages impact your pH balance just like the foods you eat. Table A-3 contains common beverages and ideas for a more alkaline-friendly exchange.

Water is typically a neutral beverage. I say *typically* because some tap water is actually acid-forming due to chemical processing. When in doubt, drink purified water, mineral water (alkaline-forming), or use a pH test strip to check your tap water.

Table A-3	Beverages
Instead of This...	*Use This...*
Black tea	Herbal tea, green tea
Coffee	Cold-pressed coffee, herbal or green tea
Fruit juice	Lemon water, unsweetened and fresh squeezed juices
Milk (cow)	Soy or almond milk
Mixed drinks (alcoholic)	Alcohol-free, sugar-free mixes and spritzers
Soda	Sparkling water

Condiments

I talk about the evils of condiments in Chapter 11, but it's important enough to get alphabetically incorporated in this appendix.

Although you may love to smother your foods with them, most condiments are overly processed, sugary concoctions that attack your pH balance. Think about why you use a condiment. Usually, it's to add flavor (or disguise flavor). The main staples on the acid alkaline diet are flavorful — hopefully you won't be trying to disguise or smother them — you'll start to enjoy their natural flavors.

I share a great recipe for alkaline-friendly "mayonnaise" in Chapter 14, which complements a sprouted grain sandwich roll or can be used as the base for creamy, homemade salad dressings.

Table A-4	Condiments
Instead of This...	*Use This...*
Ketchup	Tomato sauce (fresh, seedless pureed tomatoes) with a dash of apple cider vinegar
Mayonnaise	Almond spread, soy yogurt
Mustard (commercial)	Stone ground mustard (sugar-free)
Relish	Finely chopped cucumbers
Salad Dressing	Cold-pressed olive oil and balsamic or apple cider vinegar with a dash of pepper

Dairy

Initially, it may seem like this is the hardest food category to work around on a pH balanced diet. I can't turn a page in one of my older dog-eared cookbooks without finding a recipe riddled with cheese, cream, or egg (I also used to suffer high cholesterol — fact). Having said that, dairy is an important part of any well-balanced diet as a source of calcium and vitamin D.

If you must, you can use traditional dairy products (milk, yogurt) as your acid-forming ingredient, but be sure to always purchase no-fat versions — they're better for your heart and your pH. In the meantime, Table A-5 depicts some pH savvy ways to use the "dairy" products in your recipes.

Table A-5	Dairy Products
Instead of This...	*Use This...*
Butter	Clarified butter, olive oil
Cheese	Vegetarian cheese crumbles, fresh herbs, cheese replacement products, a sprinkle of parmesan
Cream	Almond milk, silken tofu
Eggs (whole)	Silken or crumbled tofu, egg whites (2:1 exchange for whole egg), egg replacement product
Milk	Soy or almond milk
Yogurt	Soy yogurt

Fruit

Some experts protest that you absolutely cannot eat fruit on an acid alkaline diet. Fruit contains natural sugars, which are acid-forming during digestion. However, I don't think it's healthy to discard any food group entirely, especially not this valuable source of vitamins, minerals, and fiber. Take lemons, for instance — they're one of the most alkaline-forming foods you can eat due to their high mineral content.

Some fruits are *calorie dense,* which means they have more pure sugars per bite than other fruits (think raisins as opposed to grapes). These fruits are more acid forming than others, like those that are mostly water (think watermelon). I've included the worst fruit pH offenders in Table A-6, but feel free to enjoy any fruit as long as you eat it in moderation.

Table A-6	Fruits
Instead of This...	*Use This...*
Blackberries	Blueberries
Cranberries	Strawberries
Canned in syrup	Fresh, frozen, or unsweetened canned
Dried (raisins)	Fresh or dehydrated
Oranges, tangerines	Lemons, limes
Processed (jams)	Grilled or fresh

Grains

Whole grains are an important part of your diet. I would run (not walk) from any diet that restricted my intake of whole grains. They provide loads of fiber, vitamins, and minerals that keep your body functioning at its best. Unfortunately, some grains (especially wheat) are acid forming. This includes every derivative of wheat including pasta, flour, and even commercial cereals. Never fear, there are plenty of alkaline-friendly substitutes, which are included in Table A-7.

If you're having a hard time finding alkalinizing sprouted grains (bread, bagels, tortillas), check online. Chapter 21 shows you how to shop online for some of the more hard-to-find alkaline-forming ingredients.

Table A-7	Grains
Instead of This...	*Use This...*
Breads (wheat based)	Sprouted grain bread
Buckwheat	Rolled oats, millet, spelt, quinoa
Pasta (white or wheat)	Spelt pasta or substitute pasta for grain such as quinoa
Refined flour	Almond, millet, or spelt flour
Rice (brown and white)	Wild rice, triticale, quinoa, barley, basmati rice

Meat and Other Proteins

You must have protein — there's no way around it. It's the building block of every cell in your body, from your muscles to your skin. Table A-8 displays how to substitute one meat or protein for a more alkalinizing choice in any dish.

All animal products are acid-forming to some degree. This table provides an even better choice for your pH by common protein sources. That's why you'll see poultry in both columns; skinless chicken breasts are a good substitute for steak, but firm-grilled tofu beats them both as a healthy substitute.

Be mindful of your protein serving size. Optimally, only 20 to 40 percent of your meal contains acid-forming ingredients, such as animal meat. Check out Chapter 15 if you want to see what an alkaline-forming recipe (with meat!) looks like.

Table A-8	Meat and Other Proteins
Instead of This…	*Use This…*
White fish, shellfish	Salmon, shrimp
Mussels	Clams, oysters
Red meat (beef, wild game)	Poultry, pork, seafood, tofu
Pork	Poultry, firm tofu
Poultry	Skinless, boneless poultry, tofu

Nuts and Seeds

Nuts and seeds are energy-packed sources of healthy fats, vitamins (such as E), and protein. Some of them, such as almond and pumpkin seeds, alkalinize your body during digestion. (They're also amazing in my granola recipe in Chapter 14.) Table A-9 shows which ones are better choices for your pH.

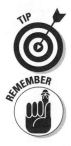

A small handful is good, otherwise it's easy to overdo it on calories. Likewise, I like to buy them in the shell. It's harder to eat too much that way.

Always reach for the raw version. Salted, roasted, and flavored nuts and seeds are usually drenched with preservatives or glazes, which combats their alkaline-forming potential.

Table A-9	Nuts and Seeds
Instead of This…	*Use This…*
Cashews	Almonds
Brazil nuts	Pine nuts, almonds
Hazelnuts	Chestnuts
Pistachios	Sunflower seeds, pumpkin seeds

Oils and Other Cooking Fats

Although most of the acid alkaline diet is fairly intuitive (animal product = bad; plant product = good), it gets tricky with oils. A few oils derived from plant sources (such as palm kernel oil) are acid-forming during digestion. Don't assume it's safe simply because it's a plant-based product.

Palm kernel oil is loaded with saturated fat, which is bad for your waistline, heart, and pH. Use Table A-10 as reference for fats to embrace and fats to avoid.

A cooking fat that's solid at room temperature is going to be acid forming. These solid fats are called *saturated fats*, which lead to high blood pressure and other heart disease.

Table A-10	Oils and Other Cooking Fats
Instead of This…	*Use This…*
Butter	Clarified butter, cold-pressed olive oil
Canola oil	Cold-pressed olive oil
Coconut oil	Clarified butter
Cooking sprays	Olive-oil-based sprays (as opposed to vegetable oil)
Lard	Coconut oil and shortening (not alkaline-forming, but better than lard)
Palm kernel oil	Avocado oil

Sweeteners

After you follow a pH-balanced diet for a while, you may notice that sweets taste sweeter and you're better able to appreciate nuances in flavors. You may even find yourself using less natural sweeteners in recipes, as your palate becomes accustomed to (and helps you appreciate) the natural flavors and subtle sugars in healthy foods.

Artificial sweeteners are abundant in many recipes, but you don't have to ditch the recipe while adhering to an alkaline diet (but please do ditch the artificial sweetener — it's so not good for you). Table A-11 gives some examples of how to substitute commercial sweeteners for more healthy options.

Table A-11	Sweeteners
Instead of This...	*Use This...*
Sugar (white, brown, raw, or confectioners)	Stevia, honey in some recipes
Artificial sweeteners	Stevia
Syrup	Organic molasses, honey

Vegetables

What? Some vegetables are acid-forming? Again, choosing a vegetable, even if it's starchy, over animal flesh or prepackaged foods is a better choice for your pH. However, some vegetables have higher sugar content and less alkaline-forming minerals than others.

The white vegetables tend to have more sugar and, therefore, negatively impact your pH (sugar = acid ash during digestion). The biggest offenders are corn and white potatoes (except for the skin, which is loaded with minerals). Table A-12 shows better veggies to choose.

Table A-12	Vegetables
Instead of This...	*Use This...*
Carrots	Beets
Corn	Eggplant, broccoli
Green beans	Asparagus
Lettuce	Spinach, endive, kale, watercress
String beans	Artichoke hearts
White potatoes	Sweet potatoes, skin of white potatoes only

Appendix B

Metric Conversion Guide

• •

*N**ote:* The recipes in this book weren't developed or tested using metric measurements. There may be some variation in quality when converting to metric units. Use the following Notes page to make your calculations.

Common Abbreviations

Abbreviation(s)	What It Stands For
cm	Centimeter
C., c.	Cup
G, g	Gram
kg	Kilogram
L, l	Liter
lb.	Pound
mL, ml	Milliliter
oz.	Ounce
pt.	Pint
t., tsp.	Teaspoon
T., Tb., Tbsp.	Tablespoon

Volume

U.S. Units	Canadian Metric	Australian Metric
¼ teaspoon	1 milliliter	1 milliliter
½ teaspoon	2 milliliters	2 milliliters
1 teaspoon	5 milliliters	5 milliliters
1 tablespoon	15 milliliters	20 milliliters
¼ cup	50 milliliters	60 milliliters
⅓ cup	75 milliliters	80 milliliters
½ cup	125 milliliters	125 milliliters
⅔ cup	150 milliliters	170 milliliters
¾ cup	175 milliliters	190 milliliters

(continued)

Volume *(continued)*

U.S. Units	Canadian Metric	Australian Metric
1 cup	250 milliliters	250 milliliters
1 quart	1 liter	1 liter
1½ quarts	1.5 liters	1.5 liters
2 quarts	2 liters	2 liters
2½ quarts	2.5 liters	2.5 liters
3 quarts	3 liters	3 liters
4 quarts (1 gallon)	4 liters	4 liters

Weight

U.S. Units	Canadian Metric	Australian Metric
1 ounce	30 grams	30 grams
2 ounces	55 grams	60 grams
3 ounces	85 grams	90 grams
4 ounces (¼ pound)	115 grams	125 grams
8 ounces (½ pound)	225 grams	225 grams
16 ounces (1 pound)	455 grams	500 grams (½ kilogram)

Length

Inches	Centimeters
0.5	1.5
1	2.5
2	5.0
3	7.5
4	10.0
5	12.5
6	15.0
7	17.5
8	20.5
9	23.0
10	25.5
11	28.0
12	30.5

Temperature (Degrees)

Fahrenheit	Celsius
32	0
212	100
250	120
275	140
300	150
325	160
350	180
375	190
400	200
425	220
450	230
475	240
500	260

Notes

Index